Child Psychopharmacology

Review of Psychiatry Series

John M. Oldham, M.D., and
Michelle B. Riba, M.D., Series Editors

Child Psychopharmacology

EDITED BY
B. Timothy Walsh, M.D.

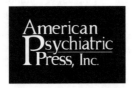

WASHINGTON, DC
LONDON, ENGLAND

Note: The authors have worked to ensure that all information in this book concerning drug dosages, schedules, and routes of administration is accurate as of the time of publication and consistent with standards set by the U.S. Food and Drug Administration and the general medical community. As medical research and practice advance, however, therapeutic standards may change. For this reason and because human and mechanical errors sometimes occur, we recommend that readers follow the advice of a physician who is directly involved in their care or the care of a member of their family.

Copyright © 1998 American Psychiatric Press, Inc.
First Edition   01   00   99   98   4   3   2
ALL RIGHTS RESERVED
Manufactured in the United States of America on acid-free paper

American Psychiatric Press, Inc.
1400 K Street, N.W.
Washington, DC   20005
www.appi.org

Library of Congress Cataloging-in-Publication Data

Child psychopharmacology / edited by B. Timothy Walsh.
     p. cm.
   Includes bibliographical references and index.
   ISBN 0-88048-833-6
   1. Pediatric psychopharmacology, I. Walsh, B. Timothy, 1946–
   [DNLM: 1. Mental Disorders—in infancy & childhood. 2. Mental
Disorders—in adolescence. 3. Mental Disorders—drug therapy.
WS 350.2 C5359 1998]
RJ504.7.C47 1998
615'.78'083—dc21
DNLM/DLC
for Library of Congress   97-52694
                                                                                        CIP

British Library Cataloguing in Publication Data
A CIP record is available from the British Library.

Contents

Contributors

F. Xavier Castellanos, M.D.   Staff Physician, Child Psychiatry Branch, National Institute of Mental Health, Bethesda, Maryland

Laurence L. Greenhill, M.D.   Associate Professor of Clinical Psychiatry, Division of Child and Adolescent Psychiatry, Columbia University College of Physicians and Surgeons; Research Psychiatrist II, New York State Psychiatric Institute; Medical Director, Disruptive Behavior Disorders Clinic, Child Psychiatry Outpatient Unit, Columbia Presbyterian Medical Center, New York, New York

Joseph Grun, B.S.   Research Assistant, Department of Child and Adolescent Psychiatry, Columbia University College of Physicians and Surgeons and New York State Psychiatric Institute, New York, New York

Sanjiv Kumra, M.D., F.R.C.P.C.   Senior Staff Fellow, Child Psychiatry Branch, National Institute of Mental Health, Bethesda, Maryland

Stan P. Kutcher, M.D., F.R.C.P.C.   Professor and Head, Department of Psychiatry, Dalhousie University; Psychiatrist in Chief, QEII Health Sciences Centre, Halifax, Nova Scotia, Canada

Laurel E. S. Mayer, M.D.   Research Fellow, Department of Psychiatry, Columbia University College of Physicians and Surgeons, New York, New York

John M. Oldham, M.D.   Director, New York State Psychiatric Institute; Professor and Vice Chairman, Department of Psychiatry, Columbia University College of Physicians and Surgeons, New York, New York

Daniel S. Pine, M.D.   Assistant Professor of Clinical Psychiatry, Department of Child and Adolescent Psychiatry, Columbia University College of Physicians and Surgeons and New York State Psychiatric Institute, New York, New York

Michelle B. Riba, M.D.   Clinical Associate Professor of Psychiatry and Associate Chair for Education and Academic Affairs, Department of Psychiatry, University of Michigan Health System, Ann Arbor, Michigan

B. Timothy Walsh, M.D.   William and Joy Ruane Professor of Psychiatry, Columbia University College of Physicians and Surgeons, New York, New York

Introduction to the Review of Psychiatry Series

John M. Oldham, M.D., and Michelle B. Riba, M.D., Series Editors

Beginning with 1998, the annual Review of Psychiatry adopts a new format. What were individual sections bound together in a large volume will be published only as independent monographs. Each monograph provides an update on a particular topic. Readers may then selectively purchase those monographs of particular interest to them. Last year, Volume 16 was available in the large volume and individual monographs, and the individually published sections were immensely successful. We think this new format adds flexibility and convenience to the always popular series.

Our goal is to maintain the overall mission of this series—that is, to provide useful and current clinical information, linked to new research evidence. For 1998 we have selected topics that overlap and relate to each other: 1) Psychopathology and Violent Crime, 2) New Treatments for Chemical Addictions, 3) Psychological Trauma, 4) Biology of Personality Disorders, 5) Child Psychopharmacology, and 6) Interpersonal Psychotherapy. All of the editors and chapter authors are experts in their fields. The monographs capture the current state of knowledge and practice while providing guideposts to future lines of investigation.

We are indebted to Helen ("Sam") McGowan for her dedication and skill and to Linda Gacioch for all of her help. We are indebted to the American Psychiatric Press, Inc., under the leadership of Carol C. Nadelson, M.D., who has supported this important and valued review series. We thank Claire Reinburg, Pamela Harley, Ron McMillen, and the APPI staff for all their generous assistance.

Foreword

B. Timothy Walsh, M.D.

In this text, which is part of the Review of Psychiatry Series, a topic of critical concern to our youngest patients and their parents is presented: the utility of medications. During the summer and fall of 1997, the *New York Times* and the *Wall Street Journal* noted the burgeoning interest of the pharmaceutical industry in the prescription of psychotropic medications for children and adolescents, and questions have been raised about whether this trend is a positive one. The chapters in this section provide clear and conservative summaries of the current state of knowledge on this topic, and they also provide guidance for the psychiatrist on the practical issues surrounding use of medication in the pediatric age range.

F. Xavier Castellanos, M.D., summarizes the pharmacological approach to tics and obsessive-compulsive disorder (OCD). Dr. Castellanos notes exciting new information suggesting that some cases of OCD may be secondary to β-hemolytic streptococcal infections. Although the importance of this etiological factor remains to be worked out, there is now little question that tics and OCD have important biological components and that there is a place for medication in their treatment.

Laurence Greenhill, M.D., reviews the treatment of attention-deficit/hyperactivity disorder (ADHD). There is more evidence supporting the utility of medication in this syndrome than for any other psychiatric disorder of childhood. Nonetheless, provocative controversies persist. Is ADHD being overdiagnosed among children? Does stimulant medication affect more than behavior in the classroom? Does ADHD disappear with maturation, or only change its presentation? Dr. Greenhill summarizes our current understanding of this extremely important area.

Work over the last 25 years has clearly established that serious disturbances of mood afflict a significant number of children and adolescents. Nonetheless, it has been surprisingly difficult to document that pharmacological interventions, which are so successful in the treatment of mood disturbances in adults, are of use in the treatment of younger individuals. Stan Kutcher, M.D., provides a concise overview of the promises and problems in this area, including recent interest in the SSRIs, which one study has found to be more effective than placebo in the treatment of major depression among children and adolescents.

Although psychosis is fortunately uncommon in childhood, its occurrence merits a careful and complete diagnostic evaluation and comprehensive treatment. Sanjiv Kumra, M.D., succinctly addresses these issues and provides a lucid summary of the benefits and side effects of antipsychotic medications in children and adolescents, including recent data on clozapine and olanzapine. Dr. Kumra's overview reflects the extensive experience of the National Institute of Mental Health (NIMH) group with the management of psychotic illness in young people and is particularly valuable, both for the information about medication and the overall management of the patient and family.

Although work on the anxiety disorders seen in children has increased substantially in recent years, controlled trials of medication are relatively few. Daniel Pine, M.D., and Joseph Grun highlight the evidence suggesting that strong links exist between anxiety disorders across the life span, and, given the paucity of data regarding the utility of medication in anxiety disorders of childhood and adolescence, summarize the most relevant data from the adult literature. Using this information, including its limitations, Dr. Pine and Mr. Grun provide useful clinical advice for incorporating medication into the treatment of anxiety disorders in children and adolescents.

Finally, Laurel Mayer, M.D., and I review current knowledge regarding the use of medication in the treatment of the eating disorders anorexia nervosa and bulimia nervosa. There has been, at most, limited progress toward developing effective pharmacological interventions for anorexia nervosa. In contrast, antidepressant medications are clearly established as being useful in the treatment of bulimia nervosa, as evidenced by the Food and

Drug Administration's (FDA's) recent approval of bulimia nervosa as an indication for fluoxetine. Unfortunately, as we emphasize, the database concerning the utility of medications for eating disorders has been derived almost entirely from studies of individuals over 18 years of age. Whether the conclusions of these studies pertain to younger patients is unknown.

Chapter 1

Tic Disorders and Obsessive-Compulsive Disorder

F. Xavier Castellanos, M.D.

Tic disorders can be severe enough to be incapacitating, but in many cases the observation of tics may serve to alert the clinician to the possible presence of other conditions that may be more impairing though not as directly observable. The best-documented comorbid diagnoses are obsessive-compulsive disorder (OCD) and attention-deficit/hyperactivity disorder (ADHD). Treatment of ADHD merits its own chapter, but the thorny issues relating to treatment of ADHD in the presence of tic disorders are included here. Although I focus exclusively on psychopharmacological interventions in this review, it should be emphasized that this approach is rarely sufficient (King and Cohen 1994; March 1995).

Definitions

DSM-IV (American Psychiatric Association 1994, p. 100) defines tics as "sudden, rapid, recurrent, nonrhythmic, stereotyped motor movement or vocalization" that may be further classified as simple or complex by comparison to prototypes. Simple tics include blinking, neck jerks, coughing, and sniffing. The prototypical complex vocal tic is coprolalia (the use of socially unacceptable words). Complex motor tics may also have an obscene content (copropraxia) but more frequently involve behaviors that may be difficult to distinguish from compulsions.

DSM-IV recognizes four types of tic disorders: Tourette's syn-

---

drome (TS), chronic motor tic (CMT) and chronic vocal tic (CVT) disorders, transient tic disorder, and tic disorder not otherwise specified.

All of the specified tic disorders require onset before age 18 years, that the disturbance not be secondary to exogenous substances or general medical conditions, and that it produce significant impairment or marked distress. TS is diagnosed when multiple motor tics and at least one vocal tic are noted frequently over a period of at least 1 year without lapses of more than 3 months. CMT and CVT have criteria that are identical to those of TS, except for the requirement that the tics be limited to motor and vocal tics, respectively. Transient tic disorder must last at least 4 weeks but no longer than 12 months.

Even more than for most psychiatric conditions, the prevalence of tic disorders varies depending on the setting, the observer, and the criteria applied. For example, in a study of 28,000 Israeli army recruits, the point prevalence of TS was 4.3/10,000 (Apter et al. 1992). However, in a more intensively studied subsample of 562 inductees (Zohar et al. 1992), the prevalence of CMT was 178/10,000. Continuity between CMT and TS is supported by studies of phenomenology (Spencer et al. 1995), familial aggregation (Pauls et al. 1990), and particularly twin studies (Hyde and Weinberger 1995), suggesting that the genetic substrates of tic disorders may be quite common (Palumbo et al. 1997).

Obsessions are defined as "persistent ideas, thoughts, impulses or images that are experienced as intrusive and inappropriate and that cause marked anxiety or distress" (American Psychiatric Association 1994, p. 418). Compulsions are defined as "repetitive behaviors (e.g., hand washing, ordering, checking) or mental acts (e.g., praying, counting, repeating words silently) the goal of which is to prevent or reduce anxiety or distress, not to provide pleasure or gratification. . . . By definition, compulsions are either clearly excessive or are not connected in a realistic way with what they are designed to neutralize or prevent" (American Psychiatric Association 1994, p. 418). However, children are not required to recognize that the obsessions or compulsions are excessive or unrealistic. It is worth noting that besides producing marked distress, obsessions or compulsions must consume at least 1 hour per day for OCD to be diagnosed. It may be testimony to the degree of distress and the predilection for record keeping and counting of OCD patients that this time criterion, unique in DSM-IV, has proven to be useful in differentiating clinical from subclinical OCD.

Comorbidity and Continuity

The development of criterion-based diagnostic systems in the 1970s and their incorporation into DSM-III in 1980 (American Psychiatric Association) marked a paradigm shift in psychiatry from which we continue to benefit. The intrinsic limits of the categorical approach have been stretched by the application of the concept of comorbidity. Thus, under our current nosology, only the rare child or adolescent presents with a single Axis I diagnosis. However, this solution may amount to sweeping unwanted complexity under the diagnostic rug. For example, children or adolescents who manifest both TS and ADHD are qualitatively distinct from children who have only TS (Schuerholz et al. 1996). Likewise, OCD symptoms in patients comorbid for TS are more likely to relate to symmetry and hoarding (Baer 1994) and to aggressive, religious, and sexual themes (Leckman et al. 1994), whereas OCD patients without TS are more likely to have symptoms focusing on contamination and cleaning.

Providing impetus for including dimensional approaches is increasing evidence that psychiatric conditions exist along continua. For example, a landmark epidemiological longitudinal study (Shaywitz et al. 1992) concluded that "reading difficulties, including dyslexia, occur as part of a continuum that also includes normal reading ability. Dyslexia is not an all-or-none phenomenon, but like hypertension, occurs in degrees. The variability inherent in the diagnosis of dyslexia can be both quantified and predicted with use of the normal-distribution model" (p. 145). The largest twin study of ADHD (Levy et al. 1997) similarly concluded "that ADHD is best viewed as the extreme of a behavior that varies genetically throughout the entire population rather than as a disorder with discrete determinants" (p. 737). Similar arguments have been constructed about tic disorders (Kurlan 1994).

A counterargument against the dimensional perspective is that the absence of clear distinctions impedes crucial decisions such as whether medical interventions are appropriate. However, the answer to this conundrum relies on the very innovation within DSM-IV that sparked controversy from investigators of the genetics of TS (Freeman et al. 1995; Kurlan 1997a)—that is, the requirement that "the disturbance cause *marked distress or significant impairment*" (American Psychiatric Association 1994, emphasis added). Since it is common for individuals in the same family to vary substantially in tic severity, this criterion complicates genetic or family studies. However, it not only serves to provide a dimensional or graded measure that determines whether an individual is a case but also provides a framework for prioritizing treatment strategies, which will be elaborated on after a brief review of theories of etiology and pathophysiology.

Etiology

The etiologies of tic disorders and OCD are still not well defined, but clear evidence exists for both genetic (Lenane et al. 1990; Walkup et al. 1996) and environmental effects, as has been elegantly delineated elsewhere (Cohen and Leckman 1994). In the early years of neuropsychiatric genetic studies (just more than a decade ago), it seemed reasonable to hypothesize that highly penetrant disorders such as TS were caused by single autosomal dominant genes (Pauls and Leckman 1986). It is now accepted that all heritable psychiatric illnesses are *complex* genetic disorders that are "caused" by an unknown number of genes interacting with each other and with undefined environmental factors.

Despite the emphasis on dimensional or graded approaches, the process of deducing biologically meaningful categories remains an important one, as illustrated by recent work on one type of immune mediation of gene-environment interactions.

A new syndrome, termed *pediatric autoimmune neuropsychiatric disorders associated with streptococcal infections* (PANDAS) (Swedo et al., in press) and characterized by prepubertal onset of OCD and/or a tic disorder with a clearly episodic course, has been proposed. The symptoms are temporally associated with group A β-hemolytic streptococcal (GABHS) infection and with neurological abnormalities such as tics, motoric hyperactivity, or choreiform movements. Choreiform movements are defined as slight and jerky irregular and arrhythmic movements of short duration that are distinct from the larger athetoid movements of Sydenham's chorea.

PANDAS may represent a *forme fruste* of Sydenham's chorea, thus providing another example of symptoms varying along a continuum yet leading to qualitative differences. Because all of the studies conducted to date with PANDAS patients have been subject to ascertainment bias, much work remains to be done to determine the prevalence of PANDAS versus nonimmune-mediated tic disorders and OCD. However, the validity of this syndrome is supported by its association with a leukocyte marker known to be associated with rheumatic fever (Murphy et al. 1997; Swedo et al. 1997) and by detection of antineuronal antibodies that cross-react with human basal ganglia in the serum of children with streptococcal-related exacerbations (Kiessling et al. 1993, 1994). At the same time, the efficacy of immune-targeting treatments for patients with PANDAS, such as intravenous infusions of immunoglobulins, plasmapheresis, or immunosuppression, has not yet been established. Until such efficacy can be demonstrated, possible cases of PANDAS with severe symptoms should be considered for referral to randomized clinical trials. Less severe cases should be treated with conventional agents, along with eradication of streptococcus, in accordance with pediatric standards of care.

Monoamines and Neuropsychiatry

PANDAS may represent the tip of a large iceberg of neuro-immune-mediated conditions that is just beginning to be explored. Clinical neuroscientists have focused for decades on the monoaminergic neurotransmitters, norepinephrine, dopamine, and serotonin. These long-favored molecules are now acknowledged to serve primarily as modulators of neurotransmission, particularly between subcortical structures and cortex. The inadequacy of animal models, our limited knowledge of the process of brain development, and the undoubted heterogeneity of our diagnostic categories all mitigate our ability to understand brain dysfunction in patients with TS, ADHD, and OCD. However, substantial advances in pharmacology have depended on manipulations of neural circuits that utilize the monoamines as their substrates. Thus, as an organizing principle, it is still useful to divide medications by their effects on one or another of these molecules. The family of serotonin selective reuptake inhibitors (SSRIs) is now the most often utilized in clinical psychiatry. Some tricyclic antidepressants (TCAs) also affect serotonin (notably clomipramine but also all tertiary amines), but all share the ability to inhibit the reuptake of norepinephrine, which is also affected by the antihypertensive agents clonidine and guanfacine. Finally, drugs that target primarily dopamine include the stimulants and neuroleptics.

The preceding statements are of course broad generalizations. All of the drugs available to us affect numerous systems, making it impossible to isolate a single system or circuit as primarily or exclusively responding to a given agent. In the same manner, diagnoses often overlap, and the three under discussion in this chapter are particularly likely to be found in combination with each other. When TS and OCD occur together, pharmacologic treatment is generally complementary. However, the combination of TS and ADHD is more problematic, because drugs that improve one group of symptoms can exacerbate the other. Thus, the discussion of TS with and without ADHD is based on the severity grid presented in Table 1–1. The diagnoses of ADHD and tic disorders form the two axes, with symptomatic severity (i.e., impairment) determining position along each axis. Since judgments of severity are necessarily doubly subjective, only three ranges are included: 1) no impairment, 2) mild to moderate impairment, and 3) marked to severe impairment. This section

Table 1–1.　Treatment of tic disorders with and without ADHD

	Mild to moderate tics	Marked to severe tics
No ADHD	1. Consider deferring drug treatment 2. Consider α_2 agonist (guanfacine or clonidine)	10. Initiate neuroleptic (haloperidol or other typical agents; pimozide; risperidone)
Mild to moderate ADHD	**Predominantly hyperactive/impulsive:** 3. Imipramine or α_2 agonist **Predominantly inattentive or combined:** 4. Methylphenidate ≤10 mg/dose 5. Methylphenidate ≤10 mg/dose + (imipramine or α_2 agonist)	**Predominantly hyperactive/impulsive:** 11. Pimozide monotherapy 12. Combination of haloperidol + (imipramine or α_2 agonist) **Predominantly inattentive or combined:** 13. Haloperidol + methylphenidate ≤10 mg/dose
Marked to severe ADHD	**Predominantly hyperactive/impulsive or combined:** 6. (Imipramine or α_2 agonist) + methylphenidate 7. Typical neuroleptic + methylphenidate **Predominantly inattentive:** 8. Methylphenidate ≤15 mg/dose 9. Methylphenidate ≤15 mg/dose + (imipramine or α_2 agonist)	**Predominantly hyperactive/impulsive:** 14. Haloperidol + imipramine or α_2 agonist **Predominantly inattentive or combined:** 15. Typical neuroleptic + methylphenidate ≤15 mg/dose 16. Typical neuroleptic + (imipramine or α_2 agonists) + methylphenidate ≤15 mg/dose

Note.　Numbered items in table respond to specific numbered points in text.

is followed by a discussion of OCD alone and in combination with the other diagnoses.

Judgments of impairment require a comprehensive biopsychosocial assessment. Such multiaxial stocktaking allows for triaging the relative importance of one diagnosis or symptom complex versus others. This process must be repeated periodically, especially to account for developmental effects that are likely to affect the priorities of symptoms. For example, tics of mild severity infrequently require treatment in elementary school children, since the child and the individuals around him or her are often unaware of the tics or their frequency. However, the same severity of tics in an adolescent may be unacceptable, thus becoming a focus of treatment.

Treatment of Tic Disorders With and Without ADHD

General Points

Dr. H. Otto Kaak, director of child psychiatry at the University of Kentucky, has taught several generations of child psychiatrists that the admonition *primum non nocere* has a corollary: "Don't just do something. Stand there!" Systematic observation is often the best initial course when assessing tic disorders and OCD, which are characterized by a waxing and waning course.

The goal of treatment of tics and OCD is to reduce symptoms to a tolerable level. Thus the symptoms producing the most distress and dysfunction must be identified and tracked.

As noted earlier, recent work on PANDAS suggests that at least some cases of neuropsychiatric illness currently diagnosable as TS and/or OCD may be caused by neuroimmune interactions with pathogenic strains of GABHS bacteria. Although controlled studies demonstrating the efficacy of invasive and noninvasive (chronic amoxicillin) therapies have not yet been completed, the well-established sequelae of streptococcal infection in vulnerable pediatric patients (those with rheumatic fever, glomerulonephritis, and Sydenham's chorea) suggest that a heightened index of suspicion for possible streptococcal involvement may be appropriate in individuals who exhibit the characteristics of PANDAS along with serological (antistreptolysin O and streptococcal antideoxyribonuclease [anti-DNase] B) or bacterial culture evidence of streptococcal exposure. At the same time, it is well known that some individuals are chronically colonized by GABHS without serological activation or morbidity. The crucial distinction is that true colonizers do not develop serological evidence of immune response. Thus, wholesale screening of children and adolescents for GABHS is not indicated.

Specific Points Referenced to Table 1–1

Point 1.   Patients with TS in the absence of other Axis I diagnoses do not differ from controls in neuropsychological function (de Groot et al. 1997; Ozonoff et al. 1994). In fact, children with TS without ADHD exceed the predicted IQs derived from parental IQ (Schuerholz et al. 1996). Thus, tics of mild to moderate severity often represent primarily a cosmetic burden that may be perceived as trivial or overwhelming, depending on the individuals and their milieu. The natural course of tic disorders is to wax and wane, with substantial amelioration by late adolescence in approximately 75% of diagnosed patients (Peterson 1996). Thus, a conservative and supportive approach may be the most appropriate.

Point 2.   The α_2 agonist clonidine was shown to be modestly effective in reducing motor tics in one influential controlled trial (Leckman et al. 1991), although significant benefit was not detected in other controlled studies (Goetz et al. 1987; Singer et al. 1995). It has been estimated that only about 25% of patients respond to clonidine (Chappell et al. 1997), but its lack of extrapyramidal symptoms (EPS), especially tardive dyskinesia (TD), has led to its continued use. Clonidine can be highly sedating, requires frequent dosing when given orally, and has rebound effects that may take months to resolve if abruptly discontinued (Leckman et al. 1986). When initiated in children, initial doses of

0.025–0.050 mg are started in the evening, with increases every 3–7 days, titrated to effect. Usual doses in elementary school children are in the range of 3–5 μg/kg/day, divided into three doses. A typical regimen after titration is 0.05 mg before school and after school, and 0.1 mg at bedtime. Some children require four doses per day; rarely, twice-daily dosing is possible. Clonidine is available as a transdermal patch that produces dermal irritation and erythema in 50% of patients. The patch is usually changed every 5 days in children instead of the 1-week interval common in adults. Safe disposal of used patches is critical.

An alternative to clonidine is guanfacine, a more specific α_2 agonist (Arnsten and Leslie 1991). In a small open-label trial, guanfacine was associated with significant improvements in motor and vocal tics and on continuous performance test (CPT) errors in doses of 0.75–3 mg/day (7 of 10 subjects took 1.5 mg) (Chappell et al. 1995). The improvement in objective testing of vigilance and impulsivity is consistent with preclinical studies (Arnsten et al. 1996). Guanfacine has a longer half-life than clonidine, allowing once-daily dosing in adults and once- or twice-daily dosing in children. The longer half-life is also associated with decreased risk of rebound hypertension (Wilson et al. 1986). Usual dosing begins with 0.5 mg once a day and titration every 3–7 days to efficacy or 3 mg/day, although one case report utilized 4 mg/day in a 6-year-old child with no adverse effects beyond initial drowsiness (Fras 1996). Balancing the potential benefits of guanfacine is the absence of controlled studies, which, however, are proceeding.

Point 3. Studies addressing the common combination of mild to moderate ADHD and mild to moderate tics using the DSM-IV distinction between inattentive and hyperactive-impulsive subtypes of ADHD have not been conducted. However, it is defensible to extrapolate from the voluminous literature on the efficacy of stimulants and TCAs in patients with ADHD, and the small but increasing literature on the same substances in TS patients.

The efficacy of TCAs in treating ADHD has been tested in 18 controlled studies (Spencer et al. 1996), with robust improvement found in behavioral symptoms in 12, moderate improvement in 5, and mixed results in 1. Since behavioral ratings are most influenced by symptoms of hyperactivity and impulsivity, it is a safe assumption that TCAs favorably affect such symptoms as defined by DSM-IV. Case reports and retrospective series (Spencer et al. 1994) and one controlled study (Singer et al. 1995) have reported that TCAs decrease tics. In the latter study, 34 children completed a double-blind crossover with fixed doses of desipramine (increasing to 25 mg qid), clonidine (increasing to 0.05 mg qid), and placebo for 6 weeks each. Desipramine was consistently superior to clonidine, showing efficacy on several measures of hyperactivity and on a global linear analog scale of tic severity, though not on clinician-rated scales. Clonidine did not demonstrate efficacy against tics on any scale, and more than two-thirds of the families in the trial requested that desipramine be continued at study conclusion. Adverse effects were more common with drug than with placebo, but no single side effect correlated significantly with a given drug. No serious adverse effects were noted in the study, which was begun before electrocardiographic (ECG) monitoring became routine for children taking TCAs. Singer and colleagues (1995) describe a reasonable regimen: "We require a normal baseline electrocardiogram or approval by a cardiologist in questionable situations, initiate desipramine at a dose not exceeding 25 mg, and gradually increase medications, if necessary, to a maximum dose of 3 mg/kg, and obtain a follow-up electrocardiogram" (p. 80).

Despite the convincing evidence of benefit from TCAs, serious concerns have arisen in recent years because of reports of sudden death among apparently healthy children taking desipramine. Although significant questions and some controversy surround this issue (Werry et al. 1995), a psychiatrist contemplating the use of a TCA in a child or adolescent is well advised to become familiar with the issues and to utilize guidelines such as those proposed by Wilens et al. (1996) (see also Chapter 4). As reflected in the practice parameters for ADHD (American Academy of Child and Adolescent Psychiatry 1997), most clinicians currently prefer imipramine or nortriptyline to desipramine. Beginning titration with 10-mg doses minimizes anticholinergic adverse effects, although constipation remains the most frequent side effect in children.

Point 4. When inattentive symptoms are prominent, low to medium doses of methylphenidate should be considered. Stimulants remain the drugs of choice for the inattentive symptoms of ADHD (see Chapter 2). However, since FDA-approved labeling for methylphenidate continues to include a boxed warning specifying that it is "contraindicated in patients who have a diagnosis or a family history of a tic disorder, including TS," a fuller discussion is necessary.

Suggestions that stimulants could cause TS (Fras and Karlavge 1977; Lowe et al. 1982) were dispelled by subsequent studies (Price et al. 1985) and clinical observations (Denckla et al. 1976), although it is generally agreed that stimulants may exacerbate tics for at least some children (Cohen and Leckman 1989; Golden 1993).

Gadow et al. (1995) examined the effect of methylphenidate in 34 boys referred primarily for treatment of ADHD with comorbid, moderately severe tics. As expected, there were robust dose-related improvements in behavior with methylphenidate (at doses of 0.1, 0.3, and 0.5 mg/kg bid), together with a "relatively benign," though statistically significant, dose-related increase in motor tic frequency on one measure during the 8-week treatment period, with no significant worsening on a dozen others. On the other hand, Riddle et al. (1995) observed a reduction in tic frequency in 5 of 5 subjects when methylphenidate was openly discontinued after an 8- to 24-month treatment period, with increases in tic frequency in 4 of the 5 when methylphenidate was resumed. My colleagues and I compared methylphenidate, dextroamphetamine, and placebo in 20 boys with ADHD and TS (Castellanos et al. 1997). At the lowest doses used in our study (15 mg methylphenidate given bid), we confirmed that stimulants did not produce statistically significant effects on ratings of tic severity (because tic severity worsened for some patients and improved for others), whereas target behaviors in the classroom improved for all. At higher doses, tic exacerbations were common and statistically significant, although this effect was often temporary with methylphenidate. Though there was one exception, tics were generally worse in patients taking dextroamphetamine during both the controlled trial and long-term follow-up. Although one-third of the subjects were not able to take stimulants long term because of intolerable effects on tics, the majority benefited, with most taking other agents in combination. We concluded that methylphenidate could be beneficial for children with ADHD and TS, although children and their parents should be advised that the scientific basis for these decisions remains scant. Importantly, we observed that stimulant-related tic exacerbations subside within several days to 2 weeks following discontinuation or dosage decrease. Consistent with sound clinical practice, the lowest effective stimulant doses should be used, since these were the least likely to produce significant increases in tic severity and no evidence of significantly increased improvement in ratings of ADHD symptoms was seen with higher doses. The tendency of methylphenidate-associated tic exacerbations to diminish over time suggests that slower increases than usual (1–2 weeks) may produce optimal improvements in ADHD symptoms with minimal worsening of TS, although this strategy was not tested.

Point 5. If low doses of methylphenidate monotherapy are insufficient to control symptoms, then adding either a TCA (Parraga et al. 1994) or α_2 agonist should be considered. The combination of clonidine and methylphenidate is currently being tested in a multisite collaborative trial. Safety concerns have been raised about this combination (Swanson et al. 1995), but closer examination of the four individual cases of death or life-threatening events did not provide "convincing evidence of any adverse interaction between clonidine and methylphenidate" (Fenichel 1995, p. 156).

Point 6. Combination therapy is generally required when symptoms of hyperactivity or impulsivity are in the marked to severe range.

Point 7. Neuroleptics carry well-known risks (Teicher and Glod 1996), but the potential benefits for patients with tics, combined with a possible improvement in symptoms of hyperactivity and impulsivity (Gittelman-Klein et al. 1976) make them an option (Shapiro and Shapiro 1981). However, haloperidol has been shown to block some of the benefits of methylphenidate in a CPT (Levy and Hobbes 1996), suggesting that this strategy has its limits.

Points 8 and 9. Doses of up to 15 mg of methylphenidate have not significantly increased tic severity in two controlled studies (Castellanos et al. 1997; Gadow et al. 1995). However, these are group results, and some individual patients experience worsening of tics at these or lower doses (Riddle et al. 1995). Thus, this higher dose range should be reserved for more severe symptoms unresponsive to low doses of methylphenidate.

Point 10. Neuroleptics are the drugs of choice for marked to severe primary tic disorders (Kurlan 1997b). For the purposes of this discussion, the three types of neuroleptics are the typical agents such as haloperidol, fluphenazine, and thiothixene; atypical neuroleptics such as risperidone; and pimozide.

Haloperidol is the most commonly prescribed typical neuroleptic for severe TS. Its advantages for pediatric use include low sedation liability, the flexibility of a liquid formulation (2 mg/ml), and "response rates approaching 80%" (Kurlan 1997b, p. 404). The initial dose of haloperidol should be 0.25 mg at bedtime, with increments of 0.25–0.5 mg every 4–7 days. The relatively long half-life allows for once-daily dosing in most cases.

With the exception of clozapine, all neuroleptics have the potential of producing EPS. However, acute EPS is most likely with high-potency agents such as haloperidol and least frequent with low-potency drugs such as thioridazine, which in turn are much more sedating. The most worrisome long-term adverse effect of typical neuroleptics, tardive dyskinesia, is uncommon in pediatric tic disorders but has been reported even with relatively low doses (Wolf and Wagner 1993). Fortunately, there have been no reports of permanent tardive dyskinesia in pediatric patients, but the symptoms lasted 4.5 years in one case (cited in Wolf and Wagner 1993). EPS and concern that tardive dyskinesia may develop are some of the factors that lead to discontinuation of neuroleptics despite efficacy in more than 80% of treated patients (Silva et al. 1996). However, other important adverse effects include dysphoric reactions, akathisia, nervousness, sedation, and "cognitive dulling/feeling drugged" (Silva et al. 1996, p. 129).

The prototypical atypical neuroleptic, clozapine, does not appear to be effective for TS (Caine et al. 1979), which is consistent with its absence of TD risk and in turn with its sparing of motor-related basal ganglia circuits (Deutch et al. 1993). It appears that D_2 blockade and EPS liability are prerequisites for neuroleptic efficacy in TS. Thus, risperidone, which was originally hoped to lack EPS and consequently have no TD risk, has been the subject of open reports describing anti-tic efficacy in adults (Bruun and Budman 1996) and children (Lombroso et al. 1995). Not coincidentally, TD has been reported after administration of risperidone in adults (Buzan 1996) and in an adolescent (Feeney and Klykylo 1996). Possible evidence of an increased EPS risk with risperidone in children and adolescents has also been noted (Mandoki 1995).

The other major adverse effect of risperidone is substantial weight gain, which averaged 8–14 pounds in one report (Lombroso et al. 1995). In another case series, 2 of 13 adolescents treated with risperidone developed fatty liver infiltration in association with marked weight gain (Kumra et al. 1997). Thus, despite its potential promise, risperidone cannot yet be considered a first-line neuroleptic for the treatment of TS pending the completion of controlled trials and more extensive documentation of its risks in youths.

The third class of neuroleptics to be discussed here has only one member, which is fitting for an agent initially approved as an orphan drug for the second-line treatment of TS. Pimozide can prolong the QT_c interval, presumably by blocking L-type calcium channels (Fulop et al. 1987). Pimozide is now contraindicated in patients receiving macrolide antibiotics such as clarithromycin, erythromycin, azithromycin, and dirithromycin, following two sudden deaths reported when clarithromycin was added to ongoing pimozide treatment ("Pimozide [Orap] contraindicated with clarithromycin [Biaxin] and other macrolide antibiotics," 1996). The presumed explanation is cytochrome P450 A3 inhibition by the macrolide, leading to toxic levels of pimozide, which can also take place when other agents such as fluoxetine are added to pimozide therapy (Ahmed et al. 1993).

Despite this drawback, the best-performed controlled trial of neuroleptics in children and adolescents with TS has found convincing evidence of the superiority of pimozide over haloperidol in anti-tic efficacy, as well as in treatment limiting adverse effects (41% with haloperidol, 14% with pimozide) (Sallee et al. 1997). On comparable doses (3.4 mg/day and 3.5 mg/day for pimozide and haloperidol, respectively), mean symptom improvement was 44% with pimozide versus 31% with haloperidol. Pimozide differed significantly from placebo on all primary and secondary tic measures, whereas haloperidol differed significantly from placebo on only one secondary measure, the Global Assessment Scale (Shaffer et al. 1983). However, pimozide did not differ significantly from haloperidol in anti-tic efficacy. Extrapyramidal symptoms were significantly more severe in patients taking haloperidol than those taking pimozide or placebo, with no significant differences seen between the latter two. Vital signs and ECG showed no significant effects. Sallee et al. (1994) concluded that neuroleptic compliance in TS could be enhanced by selecting pimozide and by limiting the dosage to less than 2 mg/day.

Point 11.   Severe TS combined with mild to moderate ADHD likely requires a combination regimen, but the possibility of monotherapy with pimozide should be explored. In an open but randomized comparison of pimozide, haloperidol, and no treatment, pimozide significantly decreased CPT commission errors in TS patients with ADHD (Sallee et al. 1994).

Point 12.   Because of the potential for life-threatening disruption of cardiac conduction, pimozide should not be combined with agents likely to interfere with its hepatic metabolism. Known inhibitors of cytochrome P450 3A3/4 include the macrolide antibiotics, fluoxetine, fluvoxamine, nefazodone, ketoconazole and other azole antifungal agents, cimetidine, and naringenin, a substance present in grapefruit (Ketter et al. 1995). Tricyclic antidepressants (Bernstein 1990) and α_2 agonists should also not be combined with pimozide to prevent cardiovascular interactions. Thus, when neuroleptic monotherapy is insufficient, haloperidol or other typical neuroleptics should be used instead.

Point 16. Although triple treatments should be reserved for the most difficult cases, we have occasionally used the combination of haloperidol, TCA or an α_2 agonist (not both), and methylphenidate (Castellanos et al. 1997).

Pharmacologic Treatment of Obsessive-Compulsive Disorder in Children and Adolescents

General Considerations

The manifestations of tic disorders and ADHD change markedly during development. By contrast, OCD symptoms, while they also fluctuate and vary within any given individual (Rettew et al. 1992), are remarkably similar across the age spectrum (March and Leonard 1996). Continuity also extends to drug response, as demonstrated by controlled studies of clomipramine (DeVeaugh-Geiss et al. 1992; Flament et al. 1985; Leonard et al. 1989) and fluoxetine (Riddle et al. 1992). All studies have demonstrated substantial amelioration of symptoms (in the range of a 50% decrease).

Continuity of drug response in the pediatric age range is particularly notable given the replicated finding that SSRI response in OCD is inversely correlated with age at onset (Ackerman et al. 1994; Ravizza et al. 1995). Thus, both studies have found that individuals "who develop the disorder later in life [after age 23 in one study] have a better chance of responding than those who become ill earlier [before age 16]" (Ackerman et al. 1994, p. 247). Further support for the relevance of age at onset comes from a study of 31 patients with childhood-onset (by age 18) OCD and/

or TS (Murphy et al. 1997). These authors found that all of the patients and only one (5%) of the healthy comparison subjects were positive for the B-lymphocyte antigen D8/17, which had previously been found to be significantly elevated in children with PANDAS (Swedo et al. 1997). Interestingly, the OCD-TS patients studied by Murphy et al. (1997) did not have an episodic course, which they defined as spontaneous remission of symptoms for at least 3 months. However, four of their patients reported "chronic waxing and waning illness with some exacerbations preceded by an acute infectious illness" (p. 405).

These intriguing studies leave many questions unanswered. How prevalent is PANDAS-related OCD compared with non-immunologically mediated varieties? Is PANDAS-related OCD less responsive to SSRIs? Can long-term antibiotic prophylaxis against streptococcal infection decrease the prevalence and incidence of these neuropsychiatric illnesses? What is the basis for the familial predisposition for streptococcus-associated autoimmune illnesses, and how is it linked to the lymphocyte antigen D8/17? Studies in progress at several centers will raise more questions as some of these answers are obtained. In the meantime, the clinician has to strike a balance that results in a sufficient index of suspicion to avoid missing severe cases of PANDAS without uncritically embracing a new perspective that might result in unnecessary treatments for children with TS or OCD. Multicenter trials have been critical for progress in pediatric medicine, and their arrival in child and adolescent psychiatry is welcome.

Practice Guidelines for OCD

To bridge the gap between research and practice, an expert consensus panel was convened by Allen Frances and colleagues to formulate guidelines for the treatment of OCD (March et al. 1997). These recommendations are also available on the World Wide Web (http://www.psychguides.com).

The guidelines for the treatment of OCD include age-specific considerations that are qualified by symptom severity. Yale-

Brown Obsessive-Compulsive Scale (YBOCS) (Goodman et al. 1989) scores of 10–18 are classified as mild OCD; YBOCS scores of 18–29 are classified as moderate and are associated with both distress and impairment; and YBOCS scores of 30 or above indicate severe OCD, with serious functional impairment. For prepubertal children, cognitive-behavioral therapy (CBT) (March et al. 1994) is recommended first, whatever the severity of OCD symptoms. Second-line treatment for prepubertal children entails the addition of a serotonin reuptake inhibitor (SRI) (i.e., the SSRIs and clomipramine, which is not selective) to CBT. The use of an SRI as the first treatment in prepubertal children is considered a second-line option.

The recommendations for adolescents with OCD vary by severity. First-line treatment for milder OCD begins with CBT alone. For more severe OCD, initiating CBT along with an SRI is recommended as the treatment of choice. Second-line treatments for milder OCD in adolescents include CBT together with SRI, or the option of starting an SRI first. For more severe OCD in adolescents, experts recommend starting either SRI or CBT alone as second-line treatments.

It is worth repeating that although the focus of this chapter is pharmacologic treatment, in prepubertal children with OCD, CBT is the consensus first choice of therapy regardless of the severity. CBT can obviously be combined with any of the medical treatments for tics or ADHD. Effective treatment of ADHD is required for effective CBT.

Serotonin Reuptake Inhibitors

An extensive review of SSRI pharmacology in children and adolescents (Leonard et al. 1997) is summarized briefly here. All SRIs are well absorbed orally, with only clomipramine undergoing extensive first-pass metabolism. Clomipramine and fluoxetine have potent metabolites; norfluoxetine's excretion half-life in adults is 7–15 days. Sertraline also has a long-lived metabolite ($t_{1/2}$ = 66 hours), although it is 5–10 times less potent than the parent compound. Since fluvoxamine and paroxetine do not have active metabolites, their abrupt discontinuation can produce unpleasant withdrawal reactions. Steady-state levels are reached in approximately 1 week for all except fluoxetine, which can take 30–90 days. Excluding fluvoxamine, all are extensively protein bound, with sertraline having the highest proportion (99%).

The popularity of the SSRIs has coincided with a heightened awareness of the importance of the cytochrome P450 system in drug kinetics and drug-drug interactions. Fluoxetine and paroxetine share the characteristics of nonlinearity at higher doses, because they inhibit both their own metabolism and that of many other drugs, including TCAs, neuroleptics, and terfenadine (Ketter et al. 1995). Fluvoxamine and sertraline are the least likely to inhibit their own metabolism and that of other drugs. None of the SSRIs should be prescribed with monoamine oxidase inhibitors (MAOIs), and the washout period with fluoxetine should be particularly lengthy (1–2 months).

The principal adverse effects of the SSRIs are behavioral: agitation, disinhibition, and akathisia. These symptoms resolve with discontinuation or decrease in dose by 50% (Riddle et al. 1991). Decreased gastric transit time can produce diarrhea or abdominal discomfort, but it generally resolves quickly if low doses are administered and increased only after steady state is reached. The availability of liquid fluoxetine makes possible the use of doses as low as 1 mg or less to start, although children with OCD, similar to affected adults, may require substantial doses after titration. Some pharmacies compound fractional doses of the other compounds. Sertraline is now available in 25-mg scored tablets, also facilitating pediatric dosing. Since these drugs are generally administered for months or years, a gradual approach is warranted.

Drug Selection

The OCD expert consensus panel did not significantly differentiate the four SSRIs from each other, although fluvoxamine and fluoxetine were the two favorites. The clear consensus is that inadequate response to one SSRI should lead to a trial of one to two other SSRIs before proceeding to the tricyclic clomipramine, which has a significantly higher response rate in meta-analyses (Greist et al. 1995), although not in head-to-head comparisons (Piccinelli et al. 1995).

When combination therapy for comorbid TS and/or ADHD is required, sertraline or fluvoxamine should be used. Even with these agents, the possibility of toxicity should be considered when evaluating potential adverse effects.

Augmentation strategies for OCD have been disappointing except when neuroleptics have been added to an SSRI for comorbid tic disorders (McDougle et al. 1994). Clonazepam augmentation of SSRI has occasionally been effective when anxiety is excessive (Leonard et al. 1994).

Conclusion

There is little doubt that the current generation of psychotropic medications has benefited many patients and their families. At the same time, substantial gaps continue to exist between our targets and our pharmacologic means. I believe that within the next one or two decades, the emerging perspectives deriving from the Human Genome Project and from molecular neuroscience will radically transform our ability to understand and ameliorate psychiatric illness. However, weighing complex options and exercising judgment with incomplete data, the art of medicine will remain necessary.

References

Ackerman DL, Greenland S, Bystritsky A, et al: Predictors of treatment response in obsessive-compulsive disorder: multivariate analyses from a multicenter trial of clomipramine. J Clin Psychopharmacol 14:247–254, 1994

Ahmed I, Dagincourt PG, Miller LG, et al: Possible interaction between fluoxetine and pimozide causing sinus bradycardia. Can J Psychiatry 38:62–63, 1993

American Academy of Child and Adolescent Psychiatry: Practice parameters for the assessment and treatment of children, adolescents, and adults with attention-deficit/hyperactivity disorder. J Am Acad Child Adolesc Psychiatry 36(suppl):85S–121S, 1997

American Psychiatric Association: Diagnostic and Statistical Manual of Mental Disorders, 4th Edition. Washington, DC, American Psychiatric Association, 1994

Apter A, Pauls DL, Bleich A, et al: A population-based epidemiological study of Tourette syndrome among adolescents in Israel. Adv Neurol 58:61–65, 1992

Arnsten AF, Leslie FM: Behavioral and receptor binding analysis of the alpha 2-adrenergic agonist, 5-bromo-6 [2-imidazoline-2-yl amino] quinoxaline (UK-14304): evidence for cognitive enhancement at an alpha 2-adrenoceptor subtype. Neuropharmacology 30:1279–1289, 1991

Arnsten AF, Steere JC, Hunt RD: The contribution of alpha 2-noradrenergic mechanisms of prefrontal cortical cognitive function: potential significance for attention-deficit hyperactivity disorder. Arch Gen Psychiatry 53:448–455, 1996

Baer L: Factor analysis of symptom subtypes of obsessive compulsive disorder and their relation to personality and tic disorders. J Clin Psychiatry 55(suppl):18–23, 1994

Bernstein M: Pimozide and tricyclics (letter). Hosp Community Psychiatry 41:454, 1990

Bruun RD, Budman CL: Risperidone as a treatment for Tourette's syndrome. J Clin Psychiatry 57:29–31, 1996

Buzan RD: Risperidone-induced tardive dyskinesia (letter). Am J Psychiatry 153:734–735, 1996

Caine ED, Polinsky RJ, Kartzinel R, et al: The trial use of clozapine for abnormal involuntary movement disorders. Am J Psychiatry 136:317–320, 1979

Castellanos FX, Giedd JN, Elia J, et al: Controlled stimulant treatment of attention-deficit/hyperactivity disorder and comorbid Tourette's syndrome: effects of stimulant and dose. J Am Acad Child Adolesc Psychiatry 36:589–596, 1997

Chappell PB, Riddle MA, Scahill L, et al: Guanfacine treatment of comorbid attention-deficit hyperactivity disorder and Tourette's syndrome: preliminary clinical experience. J Am Acad Child Adolesc Psychiatry 34:1140–1146, 1995

Chappell PB, Scahill LD, Leckman JF: Future therapies of Tourette syndrome. Neurol Clin 15:429–450, 1997

Cohen DJ, Leckman JF: Commentary on "Methylphenidate treatment of attention-deficit hyperactivity disorder in boys with Tourette's Syndrome." J Am Acad Child Adolesc Psychiatry 28:580–582, 1989

Cohen DJ, Leckman JF: Developmental psychopathology and neurobiology of Tourette's syndrome. J Am Acad Child Adolesc Psychiatry 33:2–15, 1994

de Groot CM, Yeates KO, Baker GB, et al: Impaired neuropsychological functioning in Tourette's syndrome subjects with co-occurring obsessive-compulsive and attention deficit symptoms. J Neuropsychiatry Clin Neurosci 9:267–272, 1997

Denckla MB, Bemporad JR, MacKay MC: Tics following methylphenidate administration: a report of 20 cases. JAMA 235:1349–1351, 1976

Deutch AY, Bourdelais AJ, Zahm DS: The nucleus accumbens core and shell: accumbal compartments and their functional attributes, in Limbic Motor Circuits and Neuropsychiatry. Edited by Kalivas PW, Barnes CD. Boca Raton, FL, CRC Press, 1993, pp 45–89

DeVeaugh-Geiss J, Moroz G, Biederman J, et al: Clomipramine hydrochloride in childhood and adolescent obsessive-compulsive disorder: a multicenter trial. J Am Acad Child Adolesc Psychiatry 31:45–49, 1992

Feeney DJ, Klykylo W: Risperidone and tardive dyskinesia (letter). J Am Acad Child Adolesc Psychiatry 35:1421–1422, 1996

Fenichel RR: Special communication: combining methylphenidate and clonidine: the role of post-marketing surveillance. J Child Adolesc Psychopharmacol 5:155–156, 1995

Flament MF, Rapoport JL, Berg CJ, et al: Clomipramine treatment of childhood obsessive-compulsive disorder: a double-blind controlled study. Arch Gen Psychiatry 42:977–983, 1985

Fras I: Guanfacine for Tourette's disorder (letter). J Am Acad Child Adolesc Psychiatry 35:3–4, 1996

Fras I, Karlavge J: The use of methylphenidate and imipramine in Gilles de la Tourette's disease in children. Am J Psychiatry 134:195–197, 1977

Freeman RD, Fast DK, Kent M: DSM-IV criteria for Tourette's (letter). J Am Acad Child Adolesc Psychiatry 34:400–401, 1995

Fulop G, Phillips RA, Shapiro AK, et al: ECG changes during haloperidol and pimozide treatment of Tourette's disorder. Am J Psychiatry 144:673–675, 1987

Gadow KD, Sverd J, Nolan EE, et al: Efficacy of methylphenidate for ADHD in children with tic disorder. Arch Gen Psychiatry 52:444–455, 1995

Gittelman-Klein R, Klein DF, Katz S, et al: Comparative effects of methylphenidate and thioridazine in hyperkinetic children, I: clinical results. Arch Gen Psychiatry 33:1217–1231, 1976

Goetz CG, Tanner CM, Wilson RS, et al: Clonidine and Gilles de la Tourette's syndrome: double-blind study using objective rating methods. Ann Neurol 21:307–310, 1987

Golden GS: Treatment of attention deficit hyperactivity disorder, in Handbook of Tourette's Syndrome and Related Tic and Behavioral Disorders. Edited by Kurlan R. New York, Marcel Dekker, 1993, pp 423–430

Goodman WK, Price LH, Rasmussen SA, et al: The Yale-Brown Obsessive Compulsive Scale, I: development, use, and reliability. Arch Gen Psychiatry 46:1006–1011, 1989

Greist JH, Jefferson JW, Kobak KA, et al: Efficacy and tolerability of serotonin transport inhibitors in obsessive-compulsive disorder: a meta-analysis. Arch Gen Psychiatry 52:53–60, 1995

Hyde TM, Weinberger DR: Tourette's syndrome: a model neuropsychiatric disorder (clinical conference). JAMA 273:498–501, 1995

Ketter TA, Flockhart DA, Post RM, et al: The emerging role of cytochrome P450 3A in psychopharmacology. J Clin Psychopharmacol 15:387–398, 1995

Kiessling LS, Marcotte AC, Culpepper L: Antineuronal antibodies in movement disorders. Pediatrics 92:39–43, 1993

Kiessling LS, Marcotte AC, Culpepper L: Antineuronal antibodies: tics and obsessive-compulsive symptoms. J Dev Behav Pediatr 15:421–425, 1994

King RA, Cohen DJ: The neuropsychiatric disorders: ADHD, OCD, and Tourette's syndrome, in Review of Psychiatry, Vol 13. Edited by Oldham JM, Riba MB. Washington, DC, American Psychiatric Press, 1994, pp 519–539

Kumra S, Herion D, Jacobsen LK, et al: Case study: risperidone-induced hepatotoxicity in pediatric patients. J Am Acad Child Adolesc Psychiatry 36:701–705, 1997

Kurlan R: Hypothesis II: Tourette's syndrome is part of a clinical spectrum that includes normal brain development. Arch Neurol 51:1145–1150, 1994

Kurlan R: Diagnostic criteria for genetic studies of Tourette syndrome (letter). Arch Neurol 54:517–518, 1997a

Kurlan R: Tourette syndrome: treatment of tics. Neurol Clin 15:403–409, 1997b

Leckman JF, Ort S, Caruso KA, et al: Rebound phenomena in Tourette's syndrome after abrupt withdrawal of clonidine: behavioral, cardiovascular, and neurochemical effects. Arch Gen Psychiatry 43:1168–1176, 1986

Leckman JF, Hardin MT, Riddle MA, et al: Clonidine treatment of Gilles de la Tourette's syndrome. Arch Gen Psychiatry 48:324–328, 1991

Leckman JF, Grice DE, Barr LC, et al: Tic-related vs. non-tic-related obsessive compulsive disorder. Anxiety 1:208–215, 1994

Lenane MC, Swedo SE, Leonard H, et al: Psychiatric disorders in first degree relatives of children and adolescents with obsessive compulsive disorder. J Am Acad Child Adolesc Psychiatry 29:407–412, 1990

Leonard HL, Swedo SE, Rapoport JL, et al: Treatment of obsessive compulsive disorder with clomipramine and desipramine in children
and adolescents: a double blind crossover comparison. Arch Gen
Psychiatry 46:1088–1092, 1989

Leonard HL, Topol D, Bukstein O, et al: Clonazepam as an augmenting
agent in the treatment of childhood-onset obsessive-compulsive disorder. J Am Acad Child Adolesc Psychiatry 33:792–794, 1994

Leonard HL, March J, Rickler KC, et al: Pharmacology of the selective
serotonin reuptake inhibitors in children and adolescents. J Am Acad
Child Adolesc Psychiatry 36:725–736, 1997

Levy F, Hobbes G: Does haloperidol block methylphenidate? motiva-
tion or attention? Psychopharmacology (Berl) 126:70–74, 1996

Levy F, Hay DA, McStephen M, et al: Attention-deficit hyperactivity
disorder: a category or a continuum? genetic analysis of a large-scale
twin study. J Am Acad Child Adolesc Psychiatry 36:737–744, 1997

Lombroso PJ, Scahill L, King RA, et al: Risperidone treatment of children and adolescents with chronic tic disorders: a preliminary report. J Am Acad Child Adolesc Psychiatry 34:1147–1152, 1995

Lowe TL, Cohen DJ, Detlor J, et al: Stimulant medications precipitate
Tourette's syndrome. JAMA 247:1729–1731, 1982

Mandoki MW: Risperidone treatment of children and adolescents: increased risk of extrapyramidal side effects? J Child Adolesc Psychopharmacol 5:49–67, 1995

March JS: Cognitive-behavioral psychotherapy for children and adolescents with OCD: a review and recommendations for treatment.
J Am Acad Child Adolesc Psychiatry 34:7–18, 1995

March JS, Leonard HL: Obsessive-compulsive disorder in children and
adolescents: a review of the past 10 years. J Am Acad Child Adolesc
Psychiatry 35:1265–1273, 1996

March JS, Mulle K, Herbel B: Behavioral psychotherapy for children
and adolescents with obsessive-compulsive disorder: an open trial
of a new protocol-driven treatment package. J Am Acad Child Adolesc Psychiatry 33:333–341, 1994

March JS, Frances A, Carpenter D, et al: Expert consensus treatment
guidelines for obsessive-compulsive disorder. J Clin Psychiatry
58(suppl 4):1–64, 1997

McDougle CJ, Goodman WK, Leckman JF, et al: Haloperidol addition
in fluvoxamine-refractory obsessive-compulsive disorder: a double-
blind, placebo-controlled study in patients with and without tics.
Arch Gen Psychiatry 51:302–308, 1994

Murphy TK, Goodman WK, Fudge MW, et al: B lymphocyte antigen
D8/17: a peripheral marker for childhood-onset obsessive-compulsive disorder and Tourette's syndrome? Am J Psychiatry 154:402–
407, 1997

Ozonoff S, Strayer DL, McMahon WM, et al: Executive function abilities in autism and Tourette syndrome: an information processing approach. J Child Psychol Psychiatry 35:1015–1032, 1994

Palumbo D, Maughan A, Kurlan R: Hypothesis III: Tourette syndrome is only one of several causes of a developmental basal ganglia syndrome. Arch Neurol 54:475–483, 1997

Parraga HC, Kelly DP, Parraga MI, et al: Combined psychostimulant and tricyclic antidepressant treatment of Tourette's syndrome and comorbid disorders in children. J Child Adolesc Psychopharmacol 4:113–122, 1994

Pauls DL, Leckman JF: The inheritance of Gilles de la Tourette's syndrome and associated behaviors: evidence for autosomal dominant transmission. N Engl J Med 315:993–997, 1986

Pauls DL, Pakstis AJ, Kurlan R, et al: Segregation and linkage analyses of Tourette's syndrome and related disorders. J Am Acad Child Adolesc Psychiatry 29:195–203, 1990

Peterson BS: Considerations of natural history and pathophysiology in the psychopharmacology of Tourette's syndrome. J Clin Psychiatry 57(suppl 9):24–34, 1996

Piccinelli M, Pini S, Bellantuono C, et al: Efficacy of drug treatment in obsessive-compulsive disorder: a meta-analytic review. Br J Psychiatry 166:424–443, 1995

Pimozide (Orap) contraindicated with clarithromycin (Biaxin) and other macrolide antibiotics. FDA Medical Bulletin 26:3, 1996

Price RA, Kidd KK, Cohen DJ, et al: A twin study of Tourette syndrome. Arch Gen Psychiatry 42:815–820, 1985

Ravizza L, Barzega G, Bellino S, et al: Predictors of drug treatment response in obsessive-compulsive disorder. J Clin Psychiatry 56:368–373, 1995

Rettew DC, Swedo SE, Leonard HL, et al: Obsessions and compulsions across time in 79 children and adolescents with obsessive-compulsive disorder. J Am Acad Child Adolesc Psychiatry 31:1050–1056, 1992

Riddle MA, King RA, Hardin MT, et al: Behavioral side effects of fluoxetine in children and adolescents. J Child Adolesc Psychopharmacol 1:193–198, 1991

Riddle MA, Scahill L, King RA, et al: Double-blind, crossover trial of fluoxetine and placebo in children and adolescents with obsessive-compulsive disorder. J Am Acad Child Adolesc Psychiatry 31:1062–1069, 1992

Riddle MA, Lynch KA, Scahill L, et al: Methylphenidate discontinuation and reinitiation during long-term treatment of children with Tourette's disorder and attention-deficit hyperactivity disorder: a pilot study. J Child Adolesc Psychopharmacol 5:205–214, 1995

Sallee FR, Sethuraman G, Rock CM: Effects of pimozide on cognition in children with Tourette syndrome: interaction with comorbid attention deficit hyperactivity disorder. Acta Psychiatr Scand 90:4–9, 1994

Sallee FR, Nesbitt L, Jackson C, et al: Relative efficacy of haloperidol and pimozide in children with Tourette's syndrome. Am J Psychiatry 154:1057–1062, 1997

Schuerholz LJ, Baumgardner TL, Singer HS, et al: Neuropsychological status of children with Tourette's syndrome with and without attention deficit hyperactivity disorder. Neurology 46:958–965, 1996

Shaffer D, Gould MS, Brasie J, et al: A Children's Global Assessment Scale (CGAS). Arch Gen Psychiatry 40:1228–1231, 1983

Shapiro AK, Shapiro E: Do stimulants provoke, cause, or exacerbate tics and Tourette syndrome? Compr Psychiatry 22:265–273, 1981

Shaywitz SE, Escobar MD, Shaywitz BA, et al: Evidence that dyslexia may represent the lower tail of a normal distribution of reading ability. N Engl J Med 326:145–150, 1992

Silva RR, Muñoz DM, Daniel W, et al: Causes of haloperidol discontinuation in patients with Tourette's disorder: management and alternatives. J Clin Psychiatry 57:129–135, 1996

Singer HS, Brown J, Quaskey S, et al: The treatment of attention-deficit hyperactivity disorder in Tourette's syndrome: a double-blind placebo-controlled study with clonidine and desipramine. Pediatrics 95:74–81, 1995

Spencer T, Biederman J, Wilens T: Tricyclic antidepressant treatment of children with ADHD and tic disorders. J Am Acad Child Adolesc Psychiatry 33:1203–1204, 1994

Spencer T, Biederman J, Harding M, et al: The relationship between tic disorders and Tourette's syndrome revisited. J Am Acad Child Adolesc Psychiatry 34:1133–1139, 1995

Spencer T, Biederman J, Wilens TE, et al: Pharmacotherapy of attention-deficit hyperactivity disorder across the life cycle. J Am Acad Child Adolesc Psychiatry 35:409–432, 1996

Swanson JM, Flockhart D, Udrea D, et al: Clonidine in the treatment of ADHD: questions about safety and efficacy (letter). J Child Adolesc Psychopharmacol 5:301–304, 1995

Swedo SE, Leonard HL, Mittleman BB, et al: Identification of children with pediatric autoimmune neuropsychiatric disorders associated with streptococcal infections by a marker associated with rheumatic fever. Am J Psychiatry 154:110–112, 1997

Swedo SE, Leonard HL, Mittleman B, et al: Pediatric autoimmune neuropsychiatric disorders associated with streptococcal infections (PANDAS): a clinical description of the first fifty cases. Am J Psychiatry (in press)

Teicher MH, Glod CA: Neuroleptic drugs: indications and guidelines for their rational use in children and adolescents. J Child Adolesc Psychopharmacol 1:33–56, 1996

Walkup JT, LaBuda MC, Singer HS, et al: Family study and segregation analysis of Tourette syndrome: evidence for a mixed model of inheritance. Am J Hum Genet 59:684–693, 1996

Werry JS, Biederman J, Thisted R, et al: Resolved: cardiac arrhythmias make desipramine an unacceptable choice in children. J Am Acad Child Adolesc Psychiatry 34:1239–1245, 1995

Wilens TE, Biederman J, Baldessarini RJ, et al: Cardiovascular effects of therapeutic doses of tricyclic antidepressants in children and adolescents. J Am Acad Child Adolesc Psychiatry 35:1491–1501, 1996

Wilson MF, Haring O, Lewin A, et al: Comparison of guanfacine versus clonidine for efficacy, safety, and occurrence of withdrawal syndrome in step-2 treatment of mild to moderate essential hypertension. Am J Cardiol 57:43E–49E, 1986

Wolf DV, Wagner KD: Tardive dyskinesia, tardive dystonia, and tardive Tourette's syndrome in children and adolescents. J Child Adolesc Psychopharmacol 3:175–198, 1993

Zohar AH, Ratzoni G, Pauls DL, et al: An epidemiological study of obsessive-compulsive disorder and related disorders in Israeli adolescents. J Am Acad Child Adolesc Psychiatry 31:1057–1061, 1992

Chapter 2

Attention-Deficit/ Hyperactivity Disorder

Laurence L. Greenhill, M.D.

Attention-deficit/hyperactivity disorder (ADHD) is a hetero-geneous behavioral disorder of unknown etiology that is first evident in childhood. The prevalence and chronicity of ADHD, coupled with its ability to interfere with major domains of de-velopmental relevance (Hinshaw 1994), make it a major public health concern requiring effective intervention. Clinicians are re-ferred ADHD patients of widely varying ages and stages of de-velopment. The correct identification of the ADHD patient thus requires familiarity with how the diagnosis should be estab-lished across the life span.

In this chapter, I provide a description of the DSM-IV syn-drome of ADHD (American Psychiatric Association 1994), infor-mation on prevalence, and an overview of office practice meth-ods to diagnose and treat ADHD in children.

Diagnostic and Assessment Guidelines

No single manual serves as a standard for making a diagnosis of ADHD or contains universally agreed-upon assessment meth-ods, treatments, or follow-up and monitoring procedures. In-stead, the practitioner must turn to textbooks, American Psychi-atric Association Diagnostic and Statistical Manuals (DSM), and published practice parameters from the American Academy of Pediatrics and the American Academy of Child and Adolescent Psychiatry (Dulcan 1997).

This work was supported, in part, by Grant no. 5 UO1-MH50454–02 (Dr. Greenhill) from the National Institute of Mental Health.

In the absence of common practice parameters, researchers have developed treatment algorithms for children with ADHD who enter controlled clinical trials. Such direction is found in the Medication Treatment Manual of the National Institute of Mental Health (NIMH) Multimodal Treatment Study of Attention Deficit/Hyperactivity Disorder sponsored by the U.S. Department of Education (DOE) (Greenhill et al. 1998). These treatment algorithms standardize procedures across the MTA's seven performance sites, making these guidelines relevant for office practice (Greenhill et al. 1996). In addition, diagnostic and treatment manuals have been developed for practitioners in health maintenance organizations (HMOs) (Maryary et al. 1996).

Changes in ADHD Diagnostic Criteria

The diagnosis of ADHD underwent three fundamental and marked changes, one every 7 years, between 1980 and 1994. The first stage occurred with the 1980 publication of the American Psychiatric Association's DSM-III, the first nosological effort to base the ADHD diagnosis on an impairing symptom, inattention. In so doing, it turned from the implied etiology of its former name, minimal brain dysfunction, to a more descriptive attention-deficit disorder with hyperactivity (ADDH) label. The criterion list required impairing symptoms in three dimensions: inattention (with three out of five items present), impulsivity (with three out of six items present), and hyperactivity (with two out of five items present). Subtypes included attention-deficit disorder without hyperactivity and attention-deficit disorder, residual type, for adults with the disorder.

The next version of the manual, DSM-III-R, which appeared in 1987, refined the 1980 multiple diagnostic criterion sets into a single, unweighted list of 14 items (American Psychiatric Association 1987). Symptom criteria are met only if the "behavior is considerably more frequent than that of most people of the same mental age" (p. 50). No subtypes were included, but criteria for duration and age at onset were added. The disorder had to begin before the age of 7, and the symptoms had to be present for

requires that the symptoms be present in at least two situations for the diagnosis to be made.

ADHD in Adult Patients

The prevalence of ADHD in adults and its severity and indications for treatment are unsettled issues. Although it had been assumed that children with ADHD outgrow their problems, recent prospective follow-up studies have shown that ADHD signs and symptoms may continue into adult life (American Psychiatric Association 1980). Adults with concentration problems, impulsivity, poor anger control, job instability, and marital difficulties sometimes seek help for problems they believe to be the manifestation of ADHD in adult life. Parents of children with ADHD may decide that they themselves are impaired by attentional and impulse control problems during an evaluation of their ADHD children.

The diagnosis attention-deficit disorder, residual state (ADD-R), was placed in DSM-III to cover patients over age 18 who had been diagnosed with ADD as children and were no longer motorically hyperactive but had impairment from residual impulsivity, overactivity, or inattention. The diagnosis of ADD-R was dropped from DSM-III-R. Although DSM-IV did not restore the diagnosis of ADD-R, the item lists for the ADHD syndrome are rephrased so that they can apply to adults. Furthermore, DSM-IV contains a category "in partial remission" that covers the adult with ADHD who retains some of his or her childhood ADHD problems. Finally, the category "not otherwise specified" (NOS) allows adult patients whose past childhood histories are unclear, but who have ADHD symptoms as adults, to receive a diagnosis of ADHD NOS. Such patients might not recall whether their ADHD symptoms had appeared before the age of 7 years (American Psychiatric Association Workgroup on DSM-IV 1991).

Adults with ADHD make impulsive decisions concerning their education, vocation, and personal lives that negatively affect work performance and achievement. Follow-up studies carried out by Weiss and Hechtman (1985) compared adults who had suffered from ADHD as children (index group) with adults who had no mental disorder as children (control group). The index group reported fewer years of education completed and more complaints of restlessness, sexual difficulties, and interpersonal problems. They exhibited a higher incidence of antisocial personality disorder and lower marks on clinician-rated global assessment scores. ADHD adults most often have impairment associated with attentional problems, finding it difficult to complete tasks and showing disorganization in managing long-term tasks.

Shaffer (1994), in an invited editorial, urged clinicians to exercise caution when identifying and treating adults for ADHD. First, adults cannot easily recall their own childhood history of ADHD symptoms with sufficient accuracy. The high incidence of Axis I (e.g., major depressive disorder) and Axis II (e.g., antisocial personality disorder) comorbid disorders makes it difficult to determine whether the adult's current impairment is from the comorbid condition or from the ADHD. Shaffer further notes that adult ADHD may be an infrequent condition. The one controlled prospective follow-up study with low attrition rates (Mannuzza et al. 1993) showed that only 3% of 25-year-old adults with a childhood history of ADHD had impairment related to present ADHD symptoms.

Guidelines for Treating ADHD

Fortunately, ADHD has proven to be one of the most effectively treated childhood psychiatric disorders. A quarter-century of published treatment studies and clinical experience attest to the short-term effectiveness of both behavioral and pharmacological strategies (Richters et al. 1995). It has been estimated that between 2% and 2.5% of all school-age children in North America receive some pharmacological intervention for hyperactivity (Bosco and Robin 1980), with more than 90% being treated with the psychostimulant methylphenidate (MPH) (Greenhill 1995;

Wilens and Biederman 1992). Estimates (Swanson et al. 1995b) suggest that from 1990 to 1993 the number of outpatient visits for ADHD increased from 1.6 to 4.2 million per year and the amount of MPH manufactured increased from 1,784 to 5,110 kg.

Since 1939, central nervous system stimulant drugs (amphetamines, MPH, and pemoline [PEM]) have served as a specific and effective treatment for ADHD. More than 160 controlled drug trials have established a consensus, particularly in the United States, that stimulant medications produce a robust response, reducing the symptoms of ADHD in more than 70% of school-age children (Spencer et al. 1996b). These drugs act rapidly and stop working within hours, with little carry over of effect. The short-term effects of these drugs are greater on behavior than on attention, with the average effect size on behavior almost three times that found on measures of performance (McCracken 1991; Pelham et al. 1995; Swanson 1993). However, the long-term benefit of stimulants on learning and social adjustment have not been demonstrated (Jacobvitz et al. 1990).

These effects are being studied most intensively in a large, multimodality, multisite (MTA) treatment study of ADHD. A pharmacological treatment strategy was developed in this study to standardize the stimulant treatment of children with ADHD across the MTA's seven performance sites (Greenhill et al. 1996). This protocol recommends an initial trial of the stimulants, starting with MPH doses of 5–20 mg/day, administered three times daily. If the child has prohibitive side effects or fails to benefit from the MPH, he or she is titrated on a succession of other drugs (amphetamine, PEM, and then a tricyclic antidepressant [TCA]) until a clinically meaningful response is achieved. Each of these drugs has been shown to be more effective than a placebo in double-blind, controlled drug trials. In the MTA study, approximately 77% of the 289 children randomized to MPH responded. For children who did not respond to these compounds, other medications including bupropion, venlafaxine, clonidine, and carbamazepine were used, even though they have not demonstrated clinical efficacy in controlled trials.

Behavioral programs that use contingency management programs have also proven effective (Hinshaw 1994). These treatments have short-term effects on ADHD symptoms such as gross motor overactivity, but only about half of the subjects show decreased oppositional behavior, aggression, or defiance. These treatments tend to work best in specific settings, so generalization of effect has been debated. The intensity of behavioral modification training affects outcome, as shown in studies involving parent and teacher training and peer skills and in intensive settings, such as full-day summer treatment programs (Pelham 1989; Pelham and Hoza 1987; Pelham and Murphy 1986).

The decision to treat the ADHD child with stimulants is based first and foremost on a diagnosis of ADHD. Furthermore, the ADHD symptoms must be persistent and cause functional impairment in a minimum of two settings. The child's physical examination and medical history must reveal no medical contraindication to treatment; the patient should be at least 6 years old. The administration of medication must be supervised by an adult. Both the parents and the school must be reminded that the stimulant drugs are classified as drugs of abuse, and the physician should ascertain that no relative living with the patient is currently abusing stimulants. School personnel must be willing to supervise medication administration if a pill is taken midday. These criteria are spelled out in detail in recently published practice parameters for child psychiatrists (Dulcan 1997).

Currently Approved Stimulants

Stimulants currently approved for children with ADHD include dextroamphetamine (DEX), MPH, *d,l*-amphetamine (Adderall), and magnesium PEM. Standard administration times and average dose ranges, titration schedules, and shaping of doses across the day ("sculpting") have been well described (Barkley et al. 1993; Greenhill 1995; Greenhill et al. 1996). Pharmacokinetics or pharmacodynamics of these stimulants in child patients with ADHD are also well-known (Clein and Riddle 1995; Pelham et al. 1995; Swanson et al., in press). Behavioral effects appear within 30 minutes and persist for 3–4 hours; elimination half-lives range between 2.5 (for MPH) and 12 (for PEM) hours (Clein and Riddle 1995). The concentration-enhancing and activity-reducing effects diminish greatly after the medication reaches its peak concentration in plasma, even though drug concentration can be quite high.

A voluminous pediatric psychopharmacology literature attests to the robust short-term improvements provided by stimulants in 50%–70% of children, adolescents, and adults with ADHD. Spencer and colleagues' (1996b) comprehensive review includes 161 controlled stimulant treatment studies encompassing 5 preschool, 140 school-age, 7 adolescent, and 9 adult controlled trials. Although early theorists held that the stimulants' calming effects were paradoxical and specific to school-age children with ADHD, empirical data have shown stimulants to reduce activity and lengthen sustained attention in children and college students without ADHD (Spencer et al. 1996b). If one examines only those subjects with ADHD, however, robust improvements in ADHD symptoms have been reported for adults, adolescents, and latency age children.

Spencer et al.'s (1996b) review lists only five controlled studies that exist for children under 6 years of age ($N = 144$), with robust effects reported for behavior in structured situations and on improvements in mother-child interactions. However, these reports supply too few data to determine safe dosing of stimulants for preschool children with ADHD. The fact that more than 400,000 MPH prescriptions are now being written yearly for this age group in the United States has created an urgent need for more research. Thus, the White House has listed new research on MPH for preschoolers among the top 10 priorities for medication research to be conducted by pharmaceutical companies in children.

Improvement has been reported for 65%–75% of the 5,899 patients randomized to stimulant treatment versus only 4%–30% of those assigned to placebo (Spencer et al. 1996b). Efficacy trials include 133 studies comparing MPH to placebo, 22 comparing DEX to placebo, and 6 randomized, controlled trials of PEM. Most trials have used crossover designs lasting only a few months in duration and recruited mostly Caucasian boys.

In these papers, stimulants rapidly reduced the cardinal symptoms of ADHD—impulsivity, inattention, and overactivity. Effects are cross-situational, encompassing classroom, lunchroom, playground, and home when the stimulant was given repeatedly throughout the day and in adequate dosages (Wilens and Biederman 1992). In the classroom, stimulants act on disruptive behaviors, such as interrupting and inappropriate motor activity (e.g., fidgetiness and finger tapping). When stimulant-treated ADHD children are compared to normal classroom controls, a large proportion display no clinically meaningful differences in directly observed attention (on-task behavior) or behavior, leading to the concept of "stimulant normalization" (Abikoff and Gittelman 1985). At home, stimulants improve parent-child interactions (Barkley 1988b, 1989) while increasing on-task behaviors and compliance.

Stimulants show effects across other domains. They ameliorate social skill deficits, a major area of impairment in children with ADHD. A peer-nomination study reported that stimulant treatment of boys with ADHD enhanced social standing but did not normalize peer appraisals of the boys' cooperativeness or qualities of being fun to be with (Whalen et al. 1989). MPH improves attention during baseball, so that stimulants can benefit ADHD children during organized group sports activities after school and on weekends (Pelham et al. 1990b). Stimulants address the cognitive problems often found in ADHD children by decreasing response variability and impulsive responding while increasing the accuracy of performance. They improve short-term memory (Gan and Cantwell 1982), reaction time, classroom computation (Carlson and Thomeer 1991), problem-solving games with peers (Whalen et al. 1989), and sustained attention (Matier et al. 1992). Studies of time-action stimulant effects show a different pattern of improvement for behavioral and for attentional symptoms, with behavior affected more than attention (Swanson et al., in press).

One of the most important findings is the high degree of short-term stimulant efficacy for behavioral targets, with weaker effects for cognition and learning. Large (0.8–1.0) effect sizes occur on behavioral measures, such as global improvement ratings, rating scales and checklists, and activity level in the classroom

(Kavale 1982; Ottenbacher and Cooper 1983; Thurber and Walker 1983). Smaller (0.6–0.8) effect sizes are reported on cognitive measures, including errors of omission and commission during the Continuous Performance Task (Milich et al. 1989; Schechter and Keuezer 1985).

Stimulant Effects on Comorbid Conditions

Children with ADHD commonly present with one or more Axis I comorbid disorders (Biederman et al. 1991), which may affect the response to stimulants. For example, children with comorbid anxiety disorders show an increased placebo response rate (DuPaul et al. 1994; Pliszka 1992), a greater incidence of side effects, and smaller improvements on cognitive tests (Tannock et al. 1995). Minor involuntary movements, called tics, occur in 18% of school-age children with ADHD, even when treated with placebo (Barkley et al. 1990b). Two controlled studies in children with Tourette's syndrome have shown inconsistent effects of stimulants, with some children showing worsening (Schachar et al. 1997) and others showing improving tic frequency patterns (Gadow et al. 1995). Although ADHD and mood disorders co-occur frequently, there have been no studies of stimulant effects among children with ADHD alone versus children with ADHD and depression.

The prevalence of comorbid bipolar disorder in school-age children with ADHD has been the source of much debate (Biederman, in press). Of a referred ADHD clinic population, 16% were reported to meet criteria for a mixed type of bipolar disorder, showing severe ADHD, pervasive mood dysregulation, aggressive outbursts, family dysfunction, and neuropsychological deficits (Wozniak et al. 1995). Considering the activating effects of stimulants, clinical wisdom suggests that it is best to first stabilize bipolar symptoms with lithium or valproic acid before using stimulants to control the ADHD symptoms (Biederman, in press; Spencer et al. 1996b). On the other hand, the verbal and physical aggression, negative social interactions with peers, and destruction of property found in children with comorbid conduct disorder, whether overt (Hinshaw 1994) or covert (Hinshaw et al. 1992), have been shown to respond to stimulants.

Starting Treatment With Stimulants

Reviews suggest that ADHD drug treatment research methods differ from daily office practice procedure (Jacobvitz et al. 1990). The type of drug is chosen before patients are recruited, and the dosing decisions depend on the protocol rather than on the patient's response. This approach is very different from clinical practice, where the patient's response influences these decisions. As a result, published research reports may not address the following office practice concerns (Richters et al. 1995).

Can the best dose and administration schedule of a stimulant for a particular patient be predicted by the patient's symptoms, weight, or age? Predicting drug response in an individual child is difficult. Although pretreatment patient characteristics (e.g., young age, low rates of anxiety, low severity of disorder, and high IQ) may predict a good response to MPH on global rating scales (Buitelaar et al. 1995), most research shows that no neurological, physiological, or psychological measures of functioning that are reliable predictors of response to psychostimulants have been identified (Pelham and Milich 1991; Zametkin and Rapoport 1987). Once a child responds, there is no universally agreed-upon criterion for how much the symptoms must change before the clinician stops increasing the dose. Furthermore, no standard exists for the outcome measure. For example, should global ratings alone be used, or should they be combined with more "objective" academic measures? Some have advocated a 25% reduction of ADHD symptoms, while others suggest that the dose continue to be adjusted until the child's behavior and classroom performance is "normalized."

Standard clinical practice dictates titrating stimulant medications through a standard dose range for each child but does not suggest the exact starting dose or the specific range for a particular child. The research literature suggests two divergent methods for titrating MPH for a particular child with ADHD. One is based on the child's weight, which allows one to standardize drug administration for children of different sizes. This method became popular after the publication of a seminal paper by Sprague and Sleator (1977), who reported a dissociation between the cognitive and behavioral effects of MPH. The best cognitive test performance occurred at a lower weight-adjusted dose (0.3 mg/kg), while the best behavioral response was found at a higher dose (1.0 mg/kg). Although a more recent report shows poor correlations between weight-adjusted MPH doses and the reduction of ADHD symptoms (Rapport et al. 1989), the sample size was small enough to allow for a type II error, and scrutiny of the data suggests a tendency for a weight effect. Others report the absence of correlation between weight and MPH doses chosen during open titration in a dual-site, multimodal study of ADHD. Despite its ubiquitous presence in research reports, current research does not uniformly support titrating with weight-adjusted doses.

Furthermore, the weight-adjusted titration method is problematic in office practice. Some MPH tablets are unscored, so the fractional doses (e.g., 0.3 mg/kg) demanded by this method require the pills to be cut, resulting in pill fragments of unknown strength. Weight-adjusted dose ranges (0.3 or 0.6 mg/kg/dose) may restrict a titration trial for some small children, who require higher MPH doses to treat their ADHD symptoms.

The alternative method uses fixed doses or whole MPH pills during titration. Total daily doses are increased through the 10- to 60-mg range until the child shows improvement or side effects. This escalating-dose, stepwise-titration method using whole pills reflects typical practice in the United States, as described in psychoactive drug treatment manuals (Barkley et al. 1993), in articles (Dulcan 1990; Greenhill 1995), and in continuing medical education courses offered at national meetings. However, the fixed-dose titration method may expose small children to high MPH doses, possibly resulting in untoward side effects.

The clinician also must select the best time of day for drug administration and the dose given each time. The half-lives of

MPH and DEX are quite short, and there is no evidence that the beneficial behavioral effects last after the drug is gone from the body. Dosing must be repeated during the day to cover school in the morning and homework in the afternoon. For standardization across multiple sites, research protocols prefer to limit the number of administration times and to give equal doses at each time to all children. Clinicians, on the other hand, individually adjust the timing of stimulant drug administration to each child to optimize time-response effects (Swanson et al. 1978). Clinicians often give a lower dose at the end of the day to minimize side effects (e.g., anorexia and insomnia). Other fine points of office practice—including how clinicians can teach young children to swallow pills—are not mentioned in published drug studies.

Choosing the best order and type of drug for treating a particular ADHD child. The stimulant literature does not help the clinician choose which stimulant drug is best for a particular patient, primarily because the three psychostimulants—MPH, DEX, and PEM—show equal efficacy for reducing ADHD symptoms in group studies (Pelham et al. 1990a; Wilens and Biederman 1992). Although standard preparations differ in duration of action, their long-acting forms all cover a 9-hour period (Pelham et al. 1990a). Despite the uniformity of group responses to these different medications, large differences exist in individual responses to various drugs and doses (Arnold et al. 1978; Elia et al. 1991). Therefore, the best order of their presentation for a particular patient is unknown. Furthermore, most published stimulant drug trials of children with ADHD do not indicate whether a brand or generic drug is being used.

Which ADHD symptoms should the clinician follow for determining drug responsiveness in a particular patient? Research protocols often rate the success of a drug treatment by examining changes of groups of children on different treatments rather than the individual patient. Change is measured using overall improvement on standardized rating forms, such as Clinical Global Impressions (Guy 1976). Although these global rating scales have very desirable psychometric properties—they are sensitive to medication effects (Barkley 1988a), their psychometric properties are known, normative data have been obtained, and they are used to set thresholds for inclusion in research studies—their rating scores do not always translate into reductions in specific ADHD symptoms that can be understood by parents or practitioners. Other studies monitor expensive laboratory measurements or analog classroom situations unavailable to the office practitioner (Pelham and Milich 1991). Even if the clinician were interested in using these measures, consensus is lacking about which rating form or laboratory task is best suited for clinical practice. Different studies employ different assessment, symptom monitoring, and side effect rating forms, and the rationale for selecting a particular measure is not often given.

How are stimulant drugs used to manage children with ADHD in long-term treatment? The majority of ADHD medication studies are less than 4 months long (Schachar and Tannock 1993), even though ADHD produces chronic impairment, with more than 75% of children with ADHD at age 10 continuing to meet full symptom and impairment criteria by age 15 (Barkley et al. 1990a).

Brief controlled research protocols do not include management rules for long-term clinical monitoring. Rather, research guidelines are limited to severity criteria for side effects necessary to break the blind and stop the study for a particular subject. Even if such rules are published with the findings, research reports do not state specifically how to manage mild, major, or prohibitive side effects. Nor is the clinician informed of how to handle noncompliance or the unique case. As a result, the rules that guide treatment decisions for a 6-week randomized clinical trial cannot be generalized to cover the management of drug treatment over months and years.

How the NIMH MTA study addresses these issues. The NIMH Collaborative Multisite, Multimodal Treatment Study of Children with ADHD (1992–1997) is the largest psychiatric treatment study of children with attention-deficit/hyperactivity dis-

---

order undertaken to date.[1] Its main goal is to examine the long-term effectiveness of randomly assigned treatments for ADHD over time. Although it employs sophisticated research methodology to standardize procedures across the study's many performance sites, it was designed so that its findings would be clinically relevant to practitioners and to parents.

The basic protocol is designed as a randomized clinical trial (RCT) with four treatment arms. After extensive assessments, children are randomly assigned to either a medication-only (MED) group, a behavioral-treatment-only (PSY) group, a group combining both treatments (CT), or a group referred to community practitioners after assessment (assessment and referral) (Arnold et al. 1997). The MTA's hypothesis (Richters et al. 1995) is based on a comparison across groups in children's functioning, associated comorbidities, and impairment during and after 14 months of undergoing these treatments. Five hundred and seventy-nine children with ADHD, combined subtype, ages 7–9 years, have been recruited at participating sites in the United States and Canada. Half of the sample (288 children) was randomized to treatments involving medication. The medication protocols for children randomized to the MED and CT treatment arms were identical, with the first month devoted to a titration trial for identifying each child's best dose.

The *MTA Psychopharmacology Treatment Manual* (Greenhill et

---

[1] The MTA study is a cooperative treatment study performed by six independent research teams in collaboration with the staff of the Division of Clinical and Treatment Research of the National Institute of Mental Health (NIMH), Rockville, Maryland, and the Office of Special Education Programs (OSEP) of the U.S. Department of Education (DOE). The NIMH principal collaborators are Peter S. Jensen, M.D.; L. Eugene Arnold, M.Ed., M.D.; John E. Richters, Ph.D.; Joanne B. Severe, M.S.; and Don Vereen, M.D. Principal investigators and coinvestigators from the six sites are as follows: University of California at Berkeley/San Francisco (UO1 MH50461): Stephen P. Hinshaw, Ph.D., and Glen Elliott, M.D., Ph.D.; Duke University (UO1 MH50447): C. Keith Conners, Ph.D., Karen Wells, Ph.D., and John S. March, M.D.; University of California at Irvine/Los Angeles (UO1 MH50440): James M. Swanson, Ph.D., and Dennis P. Cantwell, M.D.; Long Island Jewish Medical Center/Montreal Children's Hospital (UO1 MH50453): Howard B. Abikoff, Ph.D., and Lilly Hechtman, M.D.; New York State Psychiatric Institute/Columbia University/Mt. Sinai Medical Center (UO1 MH50454): Laurence L. Greenhill, M.D., and Jeffrey Newcorn, M.D.; University of Pittsburgh (UO1 MH50467): William E. Pelham, Ph.D., and Betsy Hoza, Ph.D. Helena C. Kraemer, Ph.D. (Stanford University), is statistical and design consultant. The principal OSEP/DOE collaborator is Ellen Schiller, Ph.D.

al. 1998) provides guidelines for the length of washout period from previous medications, choice of the order of drugs to be used, individual titration of subjects using fixed-dose methods, ranges of starting doses, types of administration schedule, choice of rating forms and symptoms rated, and emergency methods. Study clinicians use the manual to quickly determine specific management instructions for stimulant side effects or how to start a particular child on a drug using its standardized tables of doses and adjustment steps for the major medications used in treating ADHD. The manual also contains all of the MTA medication rating forms with anchor points, the scripted medication visit administration forms, and algorithms for changing doses and drugs. Standardization is enhanced by the inclusion of algorithms designed to manage changes in doses or drugs in long-term care. As a result, the MTA's medication treatment is more of a set of detailed strategies rather than instructions on how to test a single drug (Greenhill et al. 1996).

The NIMH MTA study used an elaborate double-blind, placebo-controlled method with daily dose switches of MPH for collecting dose response information on a single child. This complex design was used to standardize the determination of best MPH dose across MTA's seven widely dispersed (geographically) performance sites. It also helped control for the start-up of psychosocial treatment in the combined treatment arm when compared with the medication-only arm. Such blind titration trials have been advocated for years in the behavioral literature in the form of published guidelines for multiple-repeat, daily-switching drug assessments (Pelham and Hoza 1987; Pelham and Milich 1991). Most important for the practitioner is that the MTA titration method stipulates that each child is exposed to all of the doses in a standardized manner. In clinical practice one might stop at the first dose that provides some symptom reduction and never try a higher dose that provides optimization.

The MTA's titration trial is quite complex. A simpler method is more suitable for office practice. Instead of switching the MPH dose daily, the changes can be made on a weekly basis, with rating forms collected at the end of each week.

As in the MTA study, fixed doses should be used for titration.

One starts in a stepwise manner, with the low-dose condition being used as the child's first exposure to MPH. The low-dose MPH condition can be given on a 5 mg–5 mg–5 mg schedule (total daily dose, 15 mg). For the remaining dose conditions, the 4:00 P.M. dose is "sculpted" or set to one-half of the noon dose. Thus, the middle MPH dose condition can be given on a 10 mg–10 mg–5 mg schedule (total daily dose, 25 mg). To prevent untoward side effects in small children, the MTA protocol limits the highest MPH dose to 15 mg MPH per dose (0.8 mg/kg/dose) for those weighing 25 kg or less and is given on a 15 mg–15 mg–5 mg schedule (total daily dose, 35 mg). Larger children weighing more than 25 kg receive the 20-mg MPH condition, which is 20 mg–20 mg–10 mg (total daily dose, 50 mg). For office practice, these dose conditions can be changed once every 3–4 days in a stepwise, increasing fashion for a total initial adjustment period of 10 days. As with the MTA, doses should be given on a three-times-daily basis to cover both school and homework periods.

The MTA study advises that medication treatment should start with MPH. Short-acting MPH was chosen for the MTA study because it has more citations in the treatment literature than any other psychostimulant (Wilens and Biederman 1992); it also has the shortest half-life of the three stimulants (Birmaher and Greenhill 1989). Side effects, should they occur, are very short-lived. MPH's extremely short duration of action avoids carry-over effects that can muddy the clinician's impressions when comparing children taking different doses. Two-thirds of children with ADHD respond to MPH (Elia et al. 1991), so most of the patients started on MPH will not need to move to alternate drugs.

However, if MPH did not work, the MTA study placed the child on open titration with short-acting DEX, followed by PEM. This order is based on the number of published studies and current practice (Klein and Wender 1995; Safer et al. 1996) rather than on any clear notion of the superior efficacy of one stimulant over another. Controlled within-subject comparisons of MPH and DEX (Arnold et al. 1978; Elia et al. 1991; Pelham et al. 1990a; Winsberg et al. 1974) show that 50 out of 141 subjects did better with DEX and 37 out of 141 with MPH, the rest doing equally well with either. PEM is listed last because it has shown evidence of extremely rare hepatotoxicity, with a rate of 4 cases per 100,000 treated.

Use the CLAM and SKAMP rating forms for monitoring ADHD symptoms. Rating forms are convenient, enabling clinicians to monitor changes in an individual patient's target symptoms during repeated assessments. The MTA titration trial rating forms were based on instruments developed to be used repeatedly during the same school day. This aspect is unlike standard research ADHD symptom rating forms, which gather data on a weekly or longer basis. To assess dimensions of ADHD symptoms, the MTA used the Conners, Loney, and Milich (CLAM) Scale, a 16-item, four-point, daily rating scale that incorporates the IOWA Conners scales (Loney and Milich 1982; Pelham et al. 1989). This scale's factor structure yields information on dimensions of ADHD, including a measure of motor activity (IO), a measure of aggression (AD), and a measure of symptoms that occur in both domains (MIXED). Impairment is monitored with the modified Swanson, Kotkin, Agler, Flynn, and Pelham (SKAMP) scale (Swanson et al. 1991). This scale employs a seven-point impairment metric to track 10 different aspects of the child's daily routine. Factors include attention (AT), which highlights attention in academic settings and academic performance (DuPaul and Barkley 1990; DuPaul and Rapport 1993), and behavior (BEHAV), which tracks deportment in home and school. A third factor (INDIVIDUAL) allows parents and teachers to write in up to five target areas for improvement. During any dose adjustment period, one teacher or parent should be responsible for all of the scoring, even if other adults assist in observation.

The *MTA Psychopharmacology Manual* contains a number of specific protocols, techniques, and rating forms that were used in the study's titration phase. For example, the MTA Side Effect Rating Scales for parents and teachers can be used to monitor adverse events (AE). This slightly modified version of the Pittsburgh Side Effect Scale (Pelham 1993) uses a four-point scale ranging from 1 (none) to 4 (severe). The parents' version includes an additional item for rating insomnia. The manual provides tables that assign severity levels for each stimulant side effect (mild, major, and prohibitive) and give instructions for their management. The length of the clinician's adjustment period and open titration can be modified depending on the severity of side effects. Children with major side effects are given more time to accommodate. Finally, the manual provides a method for teaching children to swallow pills by starting with practice sessions swallowing larger and larger cake decorations.

Chronic treatment of ADHD should follow standard decision rules such as those developed for the MTA study. The MTA established a set of algorithms for managing medication decisions over the months of open medication treatment that occur in clinical practice. Decisions were based on monthly MTA Clinical Global Impression (CGI) (Guy 1976) ratings obtained from parents, teachers, and the pharmacotherapist just before or at the child's monthly appointment with the pharmacotherapist. Changes in drug or dose were controlled by algorithms based on CGI scores.

Once the child's best dose of stimulant is determined in a titration trial, no change should be allowed during the first month, other than lowering of dose for major or prohibitive side effects. After 1 month, the physician may increase the total daily MPH dose by 10 mg or total daily DEX dose by 5 mg to manage new ADHD symptoms; doses may be lowered within this range for minor side effects. Ratings of mild severity from parent, teacher, or clinician, or a single score of moderate severity or worse from any rater, suggest that an increased dose or drug change may be appropriate. If the child has major or prohibitive side effects or is nonresponsive to MPH—either during titration or during maintenance—other medications can be openly titrated and used after MPH is stopped. The MPH may be changed for new adverse events, for deterioration, and for insufficient benefit. The clinician can follow the MTA alternative-drug pharmacological algorithm, which suggests that the child be tried successively on DEX, PEM, and then a tricyclic. Efficacy studies suggest that desipramine offers the greatest efficacy in reducing the symptoms of ADHD, but safety concerns often lead clinicians to use other antidepressants, such as bupropion or imipramine, in that order.

The *Physicians' Desk Reference* suggests the top MPH doses for use in children and adolescents, which have been set at 60 mg MPH total daily dose. Recent research with adults has shown definite benefits for following a weight-adjusted (1 mg/kg/day) total daily dose, which enabled the proportion of responders in one study to reach those found in school-age children (Spencer et al. 1995). For adults, the top doses may range between 70 and 80 mg total daily dose.

Extended-Release Forms

Longer-acting stimulants, including Ritalin-SR and Dextroamphetamine Spansules, show dose equivalency and efficacy with the immediate release preparations in controlled trials of groups of ADHD children (Clein and Riddle 1995; Greenhill 1995; Greenhill et al. 1997). One study showed that PEM, DEX, and MPH long-duration preparations provided improvement for 9 hours in the cognitive but not behavioral domain (Pelham et al. 1990a). Yet longer-acting MPH-SR is perceived by clinicians as less effective for individual children (Dulcan 1990), perhaps accounting for its small market share. Promising combinations of short- and long-acting stimulant preparations have not been adequately tested in more than one controlled study (Fitzpatrick et al. 1992).

Stimulant Side Effects

Stimulants have a strong benefit-risk ratio in the pediatric age range (Klein and Wender 1995), with less than a 4% rate of severe adverse events in controlled studies (Barkley et al. 1990b). Two double-blind, placebo-controlled studies, involving 289 children with ADHD, identified five main stimulant-related side effects in children with ADHD, ages 5–15: insomnia, reduced appetite, stomachache, headache, and dizziness (Barkley et al. 1990b; DuPaul et al. 1994). ADHD children taking placebos frequently report these same physical symptoms but significantly less often than when taking active drug. On the other hand, staring, daydreaming, irritability, anxiety, and nail biting decrease with increasing stimulant dose. Behavioral rebound, motor tics, compulsive picking of nose or skin, dose-related emotional or cognitive constriction, and dose-related growth delays are not reported in placebo-controlled studies (Greenhill 1995; Spencer et al. 1996a).

Even so, clinicians are aware that the prevailing opinion that stimulant-related side effects are rare and insignificant clinically may be misleading (Schachar et al. 1997). Rates of stimulant side effects are based on short-term trials. In addition, problems with stimulant side effects may be underreported because they may be confounded with reports of poor compliance or treatment failure.

Serious late-appearing stimulant side effects have not been commonly reported, despite 30 years of extensive use among millions of children. However, public concern about MPH has been piqued by reports of rare side effects in patients, tumors in laboratory animals, and speculations fueled by substance use and abuse of related drugs, such as methamphetamine and cocaine. These side effects include stimulant-related growth delays, hepatotoxicity in children treated chronically with PEM, stimulant-related sensitization for later substance use and abuse, and altered risk of cancer based on animal studies.

One area of particular controversy is the putative growth delays from chronic stimulant treatment of growing children with ADHD. Although prospective multiyear treatment studies (Gillberg et al. 1997) have reported small weight decrements, prospective follow-up into adult life (Manuzza et al. 1991) has revealed no significant impairment of height attained. During development, however, growth curves of ADHD children, either stimulant treated or not, have demonstrated slower advances than those of normal children (Spencer et al. 1996a). Despite the increased risk for children with ADHD to become involved with substance use and abuse in adolescence, stimulant treatment has not additionally increased this risk (Loney and Milich 1982).

Two other adverse events have resulted in warnings in the stimulant's package insert, including hepatic tumors in rodents treated with high oral doses of 4–47 mg/kg of MPH (Dunnick and Hailey 1995) and for fulminant hepatotoxicity in children treated with PEM (Berkovitch et al. 1995). Hepatic tumors have not been reported in children treated with MPH. Even though the fulminant hepatotoxicity is extremely rare (occurring in no more than 4 per 100,000 children treated), PEM is no longer recommended as a first-line stimulant for ADHD treatment.

Motor or vocal tics, which appear in 1% of children taking MPH, alarm parents when they occur. A controlled trial of MPH in children with ADHD and chronic tic disorder (Gadow et al. 1995) reported significant improvement in ADHD symptoms for all subjects but no consistent worsening of tics or increase in tic frequency. However, the total daily MPH doses used never exceeded 20 mg/day. These low doses and the short 8-week study do not resemble the higher doses or longer treatment duration found in clinical practice, where tics may appear after several months of MPH administration. The clinical literature has held that MPH lowers seizure threshold, although treatment of patients with ADHD and seizures with MPH shows no change in seizure frequency (Klein and Wender 1995). As for growth, one large controlled study (Gittelman Klein et al. 1988) reported growth rate reductions among a subgroup of children, with resumption of growth immediately when treatment was interrupted (Safer et al. 1975).

Challenges of Using Stimulant Medication Treatment for ADHD

Many published clinical trials have shown that currently marketed stimulants have robust efficacy over the life span in normalizing inattentive, impulsive, and restless ADHD behaviors. This success has made it less likely for new stimulants to be developed. PEM was the last "new" stimulant to receive Food and Drug Administration (FDA) approval in the past 20 years. Although sustained-release MPH was approved in 1984 and *d,l*-amphetamine (Adderall) in 1996, both are modifications of previously available products.

Despite the enthusiasm with which they are being prescribed in the United States, stimulants are not without their problems in clinical practice. First, most immediate-release tablets have an all-too-brief 2- to 5-hour duration of action, requiring multiple doses at inconvenient times (e.g., in school). No evidence of these benefits carrying over to the next day exists. Many children experience considerable time-action effects and variability of response (Hinshaw 1994; Swanson 1993) across the school day.

Second, there is some concern that children are often medicated based on their behavior without proper regard for their cognitive responses. Studies have been mounted to evaluate the possibility that these medications may increase focus at the expense of narrowing flexibility, leading to a steadfast, rigid state that does not promote individual creativity. An early seminal study comparing responses on a paired-associate learning, short-term memory task with behavioral changes in 10 ADHD children treated with MPH suggested a dissociation of cognitive from behavioral effects and a nonlinear dose response curve in the cognitive domain (Sprague and Sleator 1977). More recent reviews of studies of cognitive functioning during stimulant treatment have objected, suggesting that MPH has linear dose-response effects on cognition, speeding response time, decreasing response variability, facilitating error detection, decreasing impulsive responding, and improving higher-order executive functions rather than just boosting lower-level processes such as encoding or memory search (Schachar et al., in press).

Third, MPH and DEX raise concerns among parents and professionals because of their Schedule II drug classification. The stimulants are grouped with agents of "high abuse potential with severe psychic or physical dependence liability" (Drug Enforcement Administration 1996) by the Drug Enforcement Administration (DEA). This action was taken 30 years ago by the DEA after learning about an epidemic of MPH use among youth in

Sweden, as well as its chemical resemblance to another drug of abuse in this country, methamphetamine. However, many years of follow-up studies, both retrospective and prospective, have yielded little hard evidence of MPH abuse by children with ADHD. Recent reports of experimentation among high school seniors and college students in the United States require more thorough investigation than the voluntary annual drug use surveys conducted among high school students.

Fourth, these drugs may show very different effects across domains (Pelham and Milich 1991), making it impossible to identify reliable predictors of drug response (Jacobvitz et al. 1990). Most of the reports of stimulant efficacy are based on short-duration, 3-month-long drug studies (Schachar and Tannock 1993) that include nonrepresentative samples of children with ADHD and use a multitude of noncomparable dosing regimens (Greenhill et al. 1996). Although pretreatment patient characteristics (young age, low rates of anxiety, low severity of disorder, and high IQ) are associated weakly with a good response to MPH (Buitelaar et al. 1995), the treatment literature has yet to describe a neurological, physiological, or psychological measure of functioning that can serve as a reliable predictor of stimulant responsivity in a given child (Zametkin and Rapoport 1987).

Fifth, there has been a perception by clinicians that some children show a loss of response to stimulants over months of treatment. Laboratory animals show tolerance to stimulant appetite-suppressing effects within 6 weeks (Cox 1990). Similarly, some children require a readjustment of dose over time, although this need is not necessarily an effect of pharmacokinetic tolerance. Other explanations for an apparent weakening of drug effect can be noncompliance with pill taking, altered caretaker expectations, growth of the child resulting in greater weight or body mass, or intercurrent stress (Dulcan 1990).

Alternative Medication Treatments

Sometimes it is best to consider using nonstimulant medications in the treatment of ADHD. Short-acting stimulants require cooperation from the school personnel for midday dosing, which may not always be possible. Stimulants, which cause insomnia, cannot be given too late in the day. MPH's attention-enhancing effects, which last only 3–4 hours, may be needed in the late evening to help school-age children with their homework, but severe insomnia may result. Several teams of investigators suggest that an unsatisfactory response to two different stimulants is required before moving on to other classes of medication (Elia et al. 1991; March et al. 1994).

The TCAs have been considered the second-line treatment for ADHD and are supported by well-designed, controlled trials of desipramine (DMI) (Biederman et al. 1989). TCAs are long acting, allow flexible dosing, and are not drugs of abuse. Dosages can be checked with plasma levels. TCAs affect cardiac conduction time, so electrocardiographic monitoring, which may be an inconvenience for families, is necessary. A series of four deaths in 1988 of ADHD children treated with DMI has made therapists cautious about its use (Werry et al. 1995), although careful statistical analyses leave uncertain whether these unfortunate occurrences were too rare to be causally linked to DMI administration (Biederman et al. 1995).

Bupropion, an antidepressant with noradrenergic activity, was reported to be effective on some of the symptoms of ADHD in placebo-controlled trials (Casat et al. 1989; Clay et al. 1988; Simeon et al. 1986). Barrickman and colleagues (1995) reported that bupropion was equivalent to MPH in the treatment of 15 children with ADHD, who showed equal improvements on both medications for the CGI, Conners teacher and parent ratings, the continuous performance test, and ratings of anxiety and depression. The study shows an order effect, which suggests a carryover from one drug condition to the next. Also, subjects were not placed on placebo in the crossover, so the study is not placebo controlled. The full results from a multisite controlled trial of bupropion (Conners et al. 1996) have now been completed and show a main effect for bupropion in reducing ADHD symptoms in the classroom.

Buspirone is an anxiolytic compound with weak dopamine (DA) activity. Current data for children with ADHD come from one small, 10-patient controlled study (McCormick et al. 1994) and case reports. One of these case reports (Quaison et al. 1991) suggests that buspirone may reduce aggressivity and ameliorate the symptoms of ADHD.

Clonidine (CLON) is an α_2-presynaptic receptor agonist indicated for adult hypertension. However, one review (Swanson et al. 1995a) reveals that there was a fivefold increase in physicians writing CLON prescriptions for children with ADHD between 1990 and 1995. These drugs have a complementary side effect profile (i.e., sedating at night, which overcomes the sleep-delaying effects of the stimulants). Safety and efficacy issues have not been addressed adequately in the pediatric age group. Only one small controlled study of 10 ADHD children (Hunt et al. 1985) suggests that CLON may be effective in ADHD, with reductions in hyperactivity and aggression. Another review (L. Williams and J. Swanson, unpublished data, December 1996) shows that publications mention only 124 CLON-treated children, 42 with ADHD, 74 with Tourette's syndrome, and 8 with early-infantile autism. Improvements average 22.9% for parent ADHD ratings in the five published studies of children with ADHD (L. Williams and J. Swanson, unpublished data, December 1996). Drug reactions including heart rate and blood pressure abnormalities have been reported for 23 children treated simultaneously with CLON and MPH. Among that group, four deaths were reported (Swanson et al. 1995a). Guanfacine, a similar α_2-presynaptic agonist, has been studied in two open trials involving 23 children (Chappell et al. 1995; Hunt et al. 1995), but no efficacy or safety data are available. Much of the popularity for the off-label use of these antihypertensives in ADHD has come from their sedating effects, useful for counteracting stimulant-related insomnia (Wilens et al. 1994).

Venlafaxine is a new antidepressant that acts as a reuptake inhibitor at both the serotonin and norepinephrine neurons. Investigators have begun reporting venlafaxine-related improvements in patients with ADHD (Adler et al. 1995; Hornig-Roher and Amsterdam 1995; Reimherr et al. 1995; Wilens et al. 1995), with symptom reductions in the 40%–60% range. Other investigators who have run small open trials with school-age children and adolescents (Luh et al. 1995; Pleak and Gornly 1995) have found that venlafaxine was well tolerated and improved ADHD symptoms. Derivan (1995), who completed a pharmacokinetic study of 25 children and adolescents with ADHD and conduct disorder, showed that these youth need a higher oral dose than adults to achieve the same blood level. He also reported improvement in CGI scores for these children and adolescents.

Selective serotonin reuptake inhibitors (SSRIs) enjoy a reputation for high efficacy and low adverse event reporting in adults with major depressive disorder. X. Castellanos (unpublished data, January 1996) found no signs of efficacy for SSRIs in the treatment of ADHD symptoms in children in the seven studies (68 children) he reviewed.

Conclusion

ADHD in children represents a panoply of challenges: for the parent, the teacher, the child, and the clinician who must make the diagnosis. By sticking close to DSM-IV and following its criteria, as well as taking a thorough history, most clinicians can gather the information necessary to make a reliable diagnosis. Brief psychopharmacological interventions with short-duration stimulant trials have been shown to have robust effects in school-age children with ADHD. Longer-term studies are needed, along with studies of preschoolers with ADHD, to show that stimulant medication treatments can be effective over the months and years required for management of chronic ADHD symptoms.

References

Abikoff H, Gittelman R: The normalizing effects of methylphenidate on the classroom behavior of ADHD children. J Abnorm Child Psychol 13:33–44, 1985

Adler L, Resnick S, Kunz M, et al: Open-label trial of venlafaxine (Effexor) in attention deficit disorder (abstract). Psychol Bull 31:544, 1995

American Psychiatric Association: Diagnostic and Statistical Manual of Mental Disorders, 3rd Edition. Washington, DC, American Psychiatric Association, 1980

American Psychiatric Association: Diagnostic and Statistical Manual of Mental Disorders, 3rd Edition, Revised. Washington, DC, American Psychiatric Association, 1987

American Psychiatric Association: Diagnostic and Statistical Manual of Mental Disorders, 4th Edition. Washington, DC, American Psychiatric Association, 1994

American Psychiatric Association Workgroup on DSM-IV: DSM-IV Options Book. Washington, DC, American Psychiatric Press, 1991

Arnold LE, Christopher J, Huestis R, et al: Methylphenidate vs. dextroamphetamine vs. caffeine in minimal brain dysfunction. Arch Gen Psychiatry 35:463–473, 1978

Arnold L, Jensen P, Richters J, et al: The National Institute of Mental Health Collaborative Multisite Multimodal Treatment Study of Children with Attention-Deficit Hyperactivity Disorder (MTA), II: methods. Arch Gen Psychiatry 37:865–870, 1997

Barkley R: Child behavior rating scales and checklists, in Assessment and Diagnosis in Child Psychopathology. Edited by Rutter M, Tuma H, Lann I. New York, Guilford, 1988a, pp 113–155

Barkley RA: The effects of methylphenidate on the interactions of preschool ADHD children with their mothers. J Am Acad Child Adolesc Psychiatry 27:336–341, 1988b

Barkley RA: Hyperactive girls and boys: stimulant drug effects on mother-child interactions. J Child Psychol Psychiatry 30:379–390, 1989

Barkley R, Fischer M, Edelbroch C, et al: The adolescent outcome of hyperactive children diagnosed by research criteria: an 8-year prospective follow-up. Journal of the American Academy of Child Psychiatry 29:546–557, 1990a

Barkley R, McMurray M, Edelbroch C, et al: Side effects of MPH in children with attention deficit hyperactivity disorder: a systematic placebo-controlled evaluation. Pediatrics 86:184–192, 1990b

Barkley R, DuPaul G, Costello A: Stimulants, in Practitioner's Guide to Psychoactive Drugs for Children and Adolescents. Edited by Werry J, Aman M. New York, Plenum, 1993, pp 205–237

Barrickman L, Perry P, Allen A, et al: A double-blind crossover trial of bupropion and methylphenidate. J Am Acad Child Adolesc Psychiatry 34:649–657, 1995

Bauermeister J, Alegria M, Bird H: Are attentional-hyperactivity deficits unidimensional or multi-dimensional syndromes? (abstract). J Am Acad Child Adolesc Psychiatry 31:423–429, 1992

Berkovitch M, Pope E, Phillips J, et al: Pemoline-associated fulminant liver failure: testing the evidence for causation (abstract). Clin Pharmacol Ther 57:696–698, 1995

Biederman J: Impact of comorbidity on the treatment of ADHD. Psychopharmacol Bull (in press)

Biederman J, Baldessarini RJ, Wright V, et al: A double-blind placebo controlled study of desipramine in the treatment of ADD, I: efficacy. J Am Acad Child Adolesc Psychiatry 28:777–784, 1989

Biederman J, Newcorn J, Sprich S: Comorbidity of attention deficit hyperactivity disorder with conduct, depressive, anxiety, and other disorders. Am J Psychiatry 148:564–577, 1991

Biederman J, Thisted R, Greenhill L, et al: Estimation of the association between desipramine and the risk for sudden death in 5- and 14-year-old children. J Clin Psychiatry 56:87–93, 1995

Birmaher BB, Greenhill L: Sustained release methylphenidate: pharmacokinetic studies in ADHD males. J Am Acad Child Adolesc Psychiatry 28:768–772, 1989

Bosco J, Robin S: Hyperkinesis: prevalence and treatment, in Hyperkinetic Children: The Social Ecology of Identification and Treatment. Edited by Whalen C, Henker B. New York, Academic Press, 1980

Buitelaar J, Gary R, Swaab-Barneveld H, et al: Prediction of clinical response to methylphenidate in children with attention deficit hyperactivity disorder. J Am Acad Child Adolesc Psychiatry 34:1025–1032, 1995

Carlson CL, Thomeer ML: Effects of Ritalin on arithmetic tasks, in Ritalin: Theory and Patient Management. Edited by Greenhill LL, Osman B. New York, Mary Ann Liebert, 1991, pp 195–202

Casat CD, Pleasants DZ, Schroeder D, et al: Bupropion in children with attention deficit disorder. Psychopharmacol Bull 25:198–201, 1989

Chappell P, Riddle M, Scahill L, et al: Guanfacine treatment of comorbid ADHD and Tourette's syndrome: preliminary clinical experience. J Am Acad Child Adolesc Psychiatry 34:1140–1146, 1995

Clay T, Gualtieri C, Evans P, et al: Clinical and neurophysiological effects of the novel antidepressant bupropion. Psychol Bull 24:143–148, 1988

Clein P, Riddle M: Pharmacokinetics in children and adolescents (abstract). Child and Adolescent Clinics of North America 4:59–75, 1995

Conners C, Casat C, Gualtieri C, et al: Bupropion hydrochloride in attention deficit disorder with hyperactivity. J Am Acad Child Adolesc Psychiatry 35:1314–1321, 1996

Cox BM: Drug tolerance and physical dependence, in Principles of Drug Action: The Basis of Pharmacology. Edited by Pratt WB, Taylor P. New York, Churchill Livingstone, 1990, pp 639–690

Derivan A, Aquir L, Preskorn S, et al: A study of venlafaxine in children and adolescents with conduct disorder (abstract). Psychopharmacol Bull 11:128, 1995

Drug Enforcement Administration conference on use of psychostimulants in the treatment of ADHD, San Antonio, TX, December 1996

Dulcan M: Using psychostimulants to treat behavior disorders of children and adolescents. Journal of Child and Adolescent Psychopharmacology 1:7–20, 1990

Dulcan M: Practice parameters for the assessment and treatment of attention-deficit/hyperactivity disorder. J Am Acad Child Adolesc Psychiatry 37:180S–190S, 1997

Dunnick J, Hailey J: Experimental studies on the long-term effects of methylphenidate hydrochloride. Toxicology 103:77–84, 1995

DuPaul GJ, Barkley RA: Medication therapy, in Attention Deficit Hyperactivity Disorder: A Handbook for Diagnosis and Treatment. Edited by Barkley RA. New York, Guilford, 1990, pp 573–612

DuPaul G, Rapport M: Does MPH normalize the classroom performance of children with attention deficit disorder? J Am Acad Child Adolesc Psychiatry 32:190–198, 1993

DuPaul G, Barkley R, McMurray M: Response of children with ADHD to methylphenidate: interaction with internalizing symptoms. J Am Acad Child Adolesc Psychiatry 33:894–903, 1994

Elia J, Borcherding B, Rapoport J, et al: Methylphenidate and dextroamphetamine treatments of hyperactivity: are there true nonresponders? Psychiatry Res 36:141–155, 1991

Fitzpatrick P, Klorman R, Brumaghim J, et al: Effects of sustained-release and standard preparations of methylphenidate on attention deficit disorder. J Am Acad Child Adolesc Psychiatry 31:226–234, 1992

Frick P, Lahey B, Appelgate B, et al: DSM-IV field trials for the disruptive and attention deficit disorders: diagnostic utility of symptoms. J Am Acad Child Adolesc Psychiatry 33:529–539, 1994

Gadow K, Sverd J, Sprafkin J, et al: Efficacy of methylphenidate for attention deficit hyperactivity in children with tic disorder. Arch Gen Psychiatry 52:444–455, 1995

Gan J, Cantwell D: Dosage effects of methylphenidate on paired associates learning: positive/negative placebo responders. J Am Acad Child Adolesc Psychiatry 21:237–242, 1982

Gillberg C, Melander H, von Knorring A, et al: Long-term central stimulant treatment of children with attention-deficit hyperactivity disorder: a randomized double-blind placebo-controlled trial. Arch Gen Psychiatry 54:857–864, 1997

Gittelman Klein R, Landa B, Mattes JA, et al: Methylphenidate and growth in hyperactive children. Arch Gen Psychiatry 45:1127–1130, 1988

Greenhill L: Attention-deficit hyperactivity disorder: the stimulants. Child and Adolescent Psychiatric Clinics 4:123–168, 1995

Greenhill L, Abikoff H, Conners CK, et al: Medication treatment strategies in the MTA: relevance to clinicians and researchers (abstract). J Am Acad Child Adolesc Psychiatry 35:444–454, 1996

Greenhill L, Halperin J, March J: Psychostimulants, in Psychiatry. Edited by Tasman A, Kay J, Lieberman J. Philadelphia, WB Saunders, 1997, pp 1659–1682

Greenhill L, Abikoff H, Arnold L, et al: Psychopharmacological Treatment Manual, NIMH Multimodal Treatment Study of Children With Attention Deficit Hyperactivity Disorder (MTA Study). Prepared by the Psychopharmacology Subcommittee of the MTA Steering Committee. Available upon request, New York, 1998

Guy W: ECDEU Assessment Manual for Psychopharmacology, Revised Edition. Washington, DC, U.S. Department of Health, Education, and Welfare, 1976, pp 287–394

Hinshaw S: Attention Deficits and Hyperactivity in Children. Thousand Oaks, CA, Sage, 1994

Hinshaw S, Heller T, McHale J: Covert antisocial behavior in boys with attention-deficit hyperactivity disorder: external validation and effects of methylphenidate. J Consult Clin Psychol 60:274–281, 1992

Hornig-Roher M, Amsterdam J: Venlafaxine versus stimulant therapy in patients with dual diagnosis of attention deficit disorder and depression (abstract). Psychol Bull 31:580, 1995

Hunt R, Minderaa R, Cohen D: Clonidine benefits children with attention deficit disorder and hyperactivity: report of a double-blind placebo-crossover therapeutic trial. J Am Acad Child Adolesc Psychiatry 24:617–629, 1985

Hunt R, Arnstan A, Asbell M: An open trial of guanfacine in the treatment of attention-deficit hyperactivity disorder. J Am Acad Child Adolesc Psychiatry 34:41–50, 1995

Jacobvitz D, Srouge LA, Stewart M, et al: Treatment of attentional and hyperactivity problems in children with sympathomimetic drugs: a comprehensive review. J Am Acad Child Adolesc Psychiatry 29:677–688, 1990

Kavale K: The efficacy of stimulant drug treatment for hyperactivity: a meta-analysis. J Learn Disabil 15:280–289, 1982

Klein R, Wender P: The role of methylphenidate in psychiatry. Arch Gen Psychiatry 52:429–433, 1995

Lahey B, Carlson C: Validity of the diagnostic category of attention deficit disorder without hyperactivity. Journal of Learning Disabilities 24:110–120, 1991

Lahey B, Appelgate B, Barkley R, et al: DSM-IV field trials for oppositional defiant disorder and conduct disorder in children and adolescents. Am J Psychiatry 151:1163–1171, 1994

Loney J, Milich R: Hyperactivity, inattention, and aggression in clinical practice, in Advances in Developmental and Behavioral Pediatrics, Vol 3. Edited by Gadow K, Bialer I. Greenwich, CT, JAI Press, 1982

Luh J, Pliszka S, Olvera R, et al: An open trial of venlafaxine in the treatment of ADHD (abstract). Psychopharmacol Bull 11:122, 1995

Mannuzza S, Klein R, Bonagura N, et al: Hyperactive boys almost grown up, V: replication of psychiatric status. Arch Gen Psychiatry 48:77–83, 1991

Mannuzza S, Klein R, Bessler A, et al: Adult outcome of hyperactive boys: educational achievement, occupational rank, and psychiatric status. Arch Gen Psychiatry 50:565–576, 1993

March J, Erhardt D, Johnston H, et al: Pharmacotherapy of attention-deficit hyperactivity disorder (abstract). Psychiatric Clin North Am 2:187–213, 1994

Maryary D, Brandt P, Koalesky A: Children With ADHD: A Manual With Decision Tree and Clinical Path. Seattle, WA, University of Washington, 1996

Matier K, Halperin J, Sharma V, et al: Methylphenidate response in aggressive and nonaggressive ADHD children: distinctions on laboratory measures of symptoms. J Am Acad Child Adolesc Psychiatry 31:219–225, 1992

McCormick L, Rizzuo G, Knickes H: A pilot study of buspirone in ADHD. Arch Gen Psychiatry 3:68–70, 1994

McCracken J: A two-part model of stimulant action on attention-deficit hyperactivity disorder in children. J Neuropsychiatry Clin Neurosci 3:201–209, 1991

Milich R, Licht B, Murphy D: Attention-deficit hyperactivity disordered boys: evaluations of and attributions for task performance on medication versus placebo. J Abnorm Psychol 98:280–284, 1989

Ottenbacher J, Cooper H: Drug treatment of hyperactivity in children. Dev Med Child Neurol 25:358–366, 1983

Pelham WE: Behavior therapy, behavioral assessment, and psychostimulant medication in the treatment of attention deficit disorders: an interactive approach, in Attention Deficit Disorder: Emerging Trends in the Treatment of Attention and Behavioral Problems in Children, Vol 4. Edited by Swanson J, Bloomingdale L. London, Pergamon, 1989, pp 169–195

Pelham W: Pharmacotherapy for children with attention-deficit hyperactivity disorder. School Psychology Review 23:199–227, 1993

Pelham WE, Hoza J: Behavioral assessment of psychostimulant effects on ADD children in a summer day treatment program, in Advances in Behavioral Assessment of Children and Families. Edited by Prinz R. Greenwich, CT, JAI Press, 1987

Pelham WE, Milich R: Individual differences in response to Ritalin in classwork and social behavior, in Ritalin: Theory and Patient Management. Edited by Greenhill LL, Osman B. New York, Mary Ann Liebert, 1991, pp 203–222

Pelham W, Murphy H: Behavioral and pharmacological treatment of hyperactivity and attention deficit disorders, in Pharmacological and Behavioral Treatment: An Integrative Approach. Edited by Hersen M, Breuning J. New York, Wiley, 1986, pp 108–147

Pelham WE, Milich R, Murphy DA, et al: Normative data on the IOWA Conners Teacher Rating Scale. Journal of Clinical Child Psychology 18:259–262, 1989

Pelham WE, Greenslade KE, Vodde-Hamilton MA, et al: Relative efficacy of long-acting stimulants on ADHD children: a comparison of standard methylphenidate, Ritalin-SR, Dexedrine spansule, and pemoline. Pediatrics 86:226–237, 1990a

Pelham WE, McBurnett K, Harper G, et al: Methylphenidate and baseball playing in ADD children: who's on first? (abstract). J Consult Clin Psychol 22:131–135, 1990b

Pelham W, Swanson J, Furman M, et al: Pemoline effects on children with ADHD: a time response by dose response analysis on classroom measures. J Am Acad Child Adolesc Psychiatry 34:1504–1514, 1995

Pleak R, Gornly L: Effects of venlafaxine treatment for ADHD in a child (letter). Am J Psychiatry 152:1099, 1995

Pliszka SR: Comorbidity of attention-deficit hyperactivity disorder and overanxious disorder. J Am Acad Child Adolesc Psychiatry 31:197–203, 1992

Quaison N, Ward D, Kitchen T: Buspirone for aggression (letter). J Am Acad Child Adolesc Psychiatry 30:1026, 1991

Rapport MD, DuPaul GJ, Kelly KL: Attention deficit hyperactivity disorder and methylphenidate: the relationship between gross body weight and drug response in children. Psychopharmacol Bull 25:285–290, 1989

Reimherr F, Hedges D, Strong R, et al: An open trial of venlafaxine in adult patients with ADHD (abstract). Psychol Bull 31:609, 1995

Richters J, Arnold L, Abikoff H, et al: The National Institute of Mental Health Collaborative Multisite Multimodal Treatment Study of Children With Attention-Deficit Hyperactivity Disorder (MTA), I: background and rationale. J Am Acad Child Adolesc Psychiatry 34:987–1000, 1995

Safer D, Allen R, Barr E: Growth rebound after termination of stimulant drugs. J Pediatr 86:113–116, 1975

Safer D, Zito J, Fine E: Increased methylphenidate usage for attention deficit hyperactivity disorder in the 1990s. Pediatrics 98:1084–1088, 1996

Schachar R, Tannock R: Childhood hyperactivity and psychostimulants: a review of extended treatment studies. Journal of Child and Adolescent Psychopharmacology 3:81–97, 1993

Schachar RJ, Ickowicz A, Tannock R: Pharmacotherapy of ADHD, in Handbook of Disruptive Behavior Disorders. Edited by Quay H, Hogan A. New York, Plenum, 1997, pp 555–565

Schachar R, Ickowicz A, Tannock R: Pharmacological treatment for attention deficit hyperactivity disorder, in New Concepts in the Study of Attention Deficit Hyperactivity Disorder. Edited by Quay H. New York, Wiley (in press)

Schechter M, Keuezer E: Learning in hyperactive children: are there stimulant-related and state-dependent effects? J Clin Pharmacol 25:276–280, 1985

Shaffer D: Attention deficit hyperactivity disorder in adults. Am J Psychiatry 151:633–638, 1994

Simeon JG, Ferguson HB, Van Wyck Fleet J: Bupropion effects in attention deficit and conduct disorders. Can J Psychiatry 31:581–585, 1986

Spencer T, Wilens T, Biederman J, et al: A double-blind, crossover comparison of methylphenidate and placebo in adults with childhood onset ADHD. Arch Gen Psychiatry 52:434–443, 1995

Spencer T, Biederman J, Harding M, et al: Growth deficits in ADHD children revisited: evidence for disorder related growth delays (abstract). J Am Acad Child Adolesc Psychiatry 35:1460–1467, 1996a

Spencer T, Biederman J, Wilens T, et al: Pharmacotherapy of attention-deficit hyperactivity disorder across the life cycle. J Am Acad Child Adolesc Psychiatry 35:409–432, 1996b

Sprague RL, Sleator EK: Methylphenidate in hyperkinetic children: differences in dose effects on learning and social behavior. Science 198:1274–1276, 1977

Swanson J: Effect of stimulant medication on hyperactive children: a review of reviews (abstract). Except Child 60:154–162, 1993

Swanson J, Kinsbourne M, Roberts W, et al: Time-response analysis of the effect of stimulant medication on the learning ability of children referred for hyperactivity. Pediatrics 61:21–29, 1978

Swanson J, Cantwell D, Lerner M, et al: Effects of stimulant medication on learning in children with ADHD. Journal of Learning Disabilities 24:219–229, 1991

Swanson J, Flockhart D, Udrea D, et al: Clonidine in the treatment of ADHD: questions about the safety and efficacy. J Child Adolesc Psychopharmacol 5:301–305, 1995a

Swanson J, Lerner M, Williams L: More frequent diagnosis of attention deficit-hyperactivity disorder (letter). N Engl J Med 333:944, 1995b

Swanson J, Wigal S, Greenhill L, et al: Adderall in children with ADHD: time-response and dose-response effects. J Am Acad Child Adolesc Psychiatry (in press)

Tannock R, Ickowicz A, Schachar R: Differential effects of MPH on working memory in ADHD children with and without comorbid anxiety. J Am Acad Child Adolesc Psychiatry 34:886–896, 1995

Thurber S, Walker C: Medication and hyperactivity: a meta-analysis. J Gen Psychol 108:79–86, 1983

Weiss G, Hechtman L: Psychiatric status of hyperactives as adults: a controlled prospective 15-year follow-up of 63 hyperactive children. J Am Acad Child Adolesc Psychiatry 24:211–220, 1985

Werry J, Biederman J, Thisted R, et al: Resolved: cardiac arryhthmias make desipramine an unacceptable choice in children. J Am Acad Child Adolesc Psychiatry 34:1239–1248, 1995

Whalen C, Henker B, Buhrmester D, et al: Does stimulant medication improve the peer status of hyperactive children? J Consult Clin Psychol 57:545–549, 1989

Wilens TE, Biederman J: The stimulants. Psychiatr Clin North Am 15:191–222, 1992

Wilens T, Biederman J, Spencer T: Clonidine for sleep disturbances associated with attention deficit hyperactivity disorder. J Am Acad Child Adolesc Psychiatry 33:424–427, 1994

Wilens T, Biederman J, Spencer T: Venlafaxine for adult ADHD. Am J Psychiatry 152:1099–1100, 1995

Winsberg BG, Press M, Bialer I, et al: Dextroamphetamine and methylphenidate in the treatment of hyperactive/aggressive children. Pediatrics 53:236–241, 1974

Wozniak J, Biederman J, Kiely K, et al: Mania-like symptoms suggestive of childhood-onset bipolar disorder in clinically referred children. J Am Acad Child Adolesc Psychiatry 43:777–786, 1995

Zametkin AJ, Rapoport JL: Neurobiology of attention deficit disorder with hyperactivity: where have we come in 50 years? J Am Acad Child Adolesc Psychiatry 26:676–686, 1987

Chapter 3

Children and Adolescents With Psychotic Disorders

Sanjiv Kumra, M.D., F.R.C.P.C.

It is now well established that schizophrenia can be diagnosed in children by the same criteria applied for adults and that autism and schizophrenia are separate disorders (J. R. Asarnow et al. 1994; Kolvin 1971; McKenna et al. 1994a; Werry and McClellan 1992). The emotional and financial burden imposed on families of children with schizophrenia is enormous. Some evidence suggests that early treatment with antipsychotic medications both decreases the immediate morbidity associated with the disorder and prevents detrimental changes that may result from prolonged untreated psychosis (Wyatt et al. 1997). The recent introduction of the "atypical" antipsychotics such as clozapine has been a major therapeutic advance for the treatment of schizophrenia (Birmaher et al. 1992; Jacobsen et al. 1994; Kowatch et al. 1995; Remschmidt et al. 1994; Towbin et al. 1993). Whether these drugs will also benefit children with other psychotic disorders is currently unknown.

The article "Practice Parameters for the Assessment and Treatment of Children and Adolescents with Schizophrenia" was published by the *American Academy of Child and Adolescent Psychiatry* (McClellan and Werry 1994; McClellan et al. 1997). In this

I would like to thank the following staff members who cared for the patients in the Childhood-Onset Schizophrenia Project and/or assisted in the preparation of this manuscript: Drs. C. T. Gordon, Kathleen McKenna, Jean Frazier, and Leslie Jacobsen; Marge Lenane, L.I.C.S.W.; Claudia Briguglio, R.N., M.N.; Ingrid Hope, M.S.N.; Mary McMahanon, R.N., M.S.N.; Lisa Hodges, R.N., M.S.; Lynn Compton, R.N.; Gail Butterworth, R.N., M.A.; and the nurses of the Child Psychiatry Branch; as well as Phyllis Siegrist, M.A.Ed.; Anna Davidson, M.Ed.; Edythe Wiggs, Ph.D.; Robin Greenfield, C.T.R.S.; Dale R. Grothe, Pharm.D., B.C.P.P.; Marcia Smith, C.T.R.S.; Thomas Fernandez, B.A.; Jeffrey Bedwell, B.S.; and Susan Gardner, M.S., O.T.R./L.

chapter, I focus primarily on research conducted since those publications. The outline of this chapter has been adapted from the recently published article "Practice Guideline for the Treatment of Patients With Schizophrenia" (for adults) (American Psychiatric Association 1997). The reader is referred to these papers and other sources (M. Campbell and Cueva 1995a, 1995b, in press; Volkmar 1996) for additional information regarding the care of children and adolescents with psychotic disorders. This chapter is divided in three sections: 1) the clinical and neurobiological aspects of childhood-onset psychotic disorders, 2) the general principles of treatment, and 3) an overview of antipsychotic treatments.

Clinical and Neurobiological Aspects of Childhood-Onset Psychotic Disorders

Childhood-Onset Schizophrenia

Childhood-onset schizophrenia (onset of psychotic symptoms before age 12) is a severe form of schizophrenia with a treated prevalence almost 50 times less frequent than the prevalence for adults (Beitchman 1985). The few studies to examine the phenomenology of childhood-onset schizophrenia (COS) using DSM-III (American Psychiatric Association 1980) criteria (Cantor et al. 1982; W. H. Green et al. 1992; Russell et al. 1989) support phenomenologic continuity with later-onset schizophrenia.

Schizophrenia in children is frequently insidious rather than acute in onset, and the most commonly reported psychotic features reported by patients are auditory hallucinations and delusions (W. H. Green et al. 1992; Kolvin 1971; Russell et al. 1989). The presence of formal thought disorder, however, is more variable and depends on the sample, and there is little agreement on how to describe the speech of children with COS (Caplan 1994). Specifically, terms used to describe thought disorder such as *illogicality, loose associations, tangentiality,* and *poverty* have been used very differently by different clinicians (Caplan 1994). During adolescence the frequency of psychotic illness increases markedly, and symptomatology is generally similar to that of adults, likely reflecting increased cognitive abilities (Hafner and Nowotny 1995; Hafner et al. 1995; Makowski et al. 1997; Schulz 1997).

The nature of the psychological and neurobiological processes underlying COS has been an important research topic. Neurobiological studies of COS patients have supported continuity with adult schizophrenia on such disparate measures as smooth-pursuit eye tracking, autonomic activity, persistence of subtle neurological signs, neuropsychological testing, anatomic brain magnetic resonance imaging (MRI), and proton magnetic resonance spectroscopy (Jacobsen and Rapoport, in press). Similar to adult-onset schizophrenia, the majority of pediatric patients experience chronic disability and significant deterioration in adaptive function from already impaired premorbid levels (Werry et al. 1991). In one study, despite extensive pharmacologic and psychosocial treatment, approximately two-thirds of patients continued to present with schizophrenia at 2- to 7-year follow-ups (J. R. Asarnow et al. 1994). Premorbid function appears to be the best predictor of clinical outcome (Werry and McClellan 1992).

In contrast to adult schizophrenia, there appears to be a high rate of cytogenetic abnormalities in patients with COS. In a group of treatment-refractory COS patients, 3 out of 38 (7.9%) subjects were found to have cytogenetic abnormalities: a case of a 1:7 translocation, a case of a 22q11 deletion or velo-cardiofacial syndrome, and a case of a 45, XO mosaic (Gordon et al. 1994; Kumra et al., in press [a]; Yan et al., in press). In addition, preliminary longitudinal data suggest a more dynamic ongoing pathophysiologic process after onset of psychosis in COS as indicated by progressive changes in brain morphology (Jacobsen and Rapoport, in press; Rapoport et al. 1997).

Diagnostic assessment. The assessment of a child or adolescent with possible psychosis involves obtaining a careful history and assessment of mental status over multiple sessions. Collateral data should be obtained, and other specialists (e.g., school reports, previous neuropsychological test data, speech and language evaluations, and neurological and genetics consultations) consulted. To prevent misdiagnosis, each child or adolescent with a diagnosis of schizophrenia should be followed closely for several years (Werry et al. 1991).

As suggested by McClellan and Werry (1994), a developmental history is important as part of the evaluation of COS and other childhood psychotic disorders. Follow-back studies tend to suggest that before the appearance of schizophrenic symptoms, precursors of the disorder may include developmental delays, disruptive behavior disorders, expressive and receptive language deficits, impaired gross motor functioning, learning and academic problems, full-scale IQ in the borderline to low-average range, and transient symptoms of pervasive developmental disorder (Alaghband-Rad et al. 1995; Russell et al. 1989; Watkins et al. 1988; Werry et al. 1991). Although similar premorbid abnormalities have been observed in patients with adult-onset schizophrenia (Crow et al. 1995; Parnas et al. 1982; Walker et al. 1994), the rate of language impairments and transient autistic-like symptoms appears higher in COS (Hollis 1995).

Since the diagnosis of schizophrenia carries specific treatment and prognostic implications, diagnostic accuracy is of considerable importance. Unfortunately, the term *childhood-onset schizophrenia* has been used overinclusively in the past to describe a broad range of severely disturbed children with some psychotic symptoms (McKenna et al. 1994a). To help make the diagnosis, information about the onset of the condition, changes in academic and social functioning, and developmental and family history should be sought. It should be stressed that evidence of both social impairment and chronicity are required to make a diagnosis of schizophrenia and that the presence of hallucinations and delusions alone does not always indicate a diagnosis of schizophrenia, since these symptoms are commonly observed in patients with affective psychoses (Werry et al. 1991).

Children With Psychotic Disorder Not Otherwise Specified

It has been well recognized by child psychiatrists that a considerable group of children with complex developmental disorders and brief "psychotic" symptoms fall outside of current syndrome boundaries (Cantor et al. 1982; Cohen et al. 1986; Greenman et al. 1986; Lofgren et al. 1991; McKenna et al. 1994a; Towbin et al. 1993; Van Der Gaag et al. 1995). These children have been given various labels such as borderline and multiplex developmental disorder (MDD) to emphasize the developmental nature of their difficulties (Greenman et al. 1986; Towbin et al. 1993). Because of the clinical heterogeneity of this group, we chose to narrowly define a subgroup from this population whom we provisionally labeled as multidimensionally impaired (MDI) (Gordon et al. 1994; Kumra et al. 1998a; McKenna et al. 1994a, 1994b). MDI children can be reliably diagnosed using empirically derived criteria (kappa of 0.81) (McKenna et al. 1994a).

Both MDI and MDD children are characterized by brief psychotic symptoms (e.g., poor ability to distinguish fantasy from reality and perceptual disturbances), prominent attention and impulse control difficulties, and nearly daily periods of emotional lability disproportionate to precipitants (Gordon et al. 1994; Towbin et al. 1993). In addition, both disorders are associated with an overrepresentation of male subjects, onset of cognitive and behavior difficulties before age 7, treatment refractoriness, poor interpersonal skills despite a desire to initiate social interactions with peers, and increased rates of schizophrenia-spectrum disorders in first-degree relatives (Kumra et al. 1998a). The rate of sex chromosome aneuploidies in MDI children (11%) was found to be higher than the rate in children with mild mental retardation (Kumra et al., in press [a]). Children with MDI or MDD differ from children within the pervasive developmental disorder spectrum in terms of their imaginative play interests, preserved social relatedness, psychotic thinking, and inconsistent level of functioning (Kumra et al. 1998a; Towbin et al. 1993; Van Der Gaag et al. 1995).

Children with MDI resemble their COS counterparts in terms of a similar pattern of premorbid developmental difficulties, information processing deficits, and brain MRI abnormalities (Kumra et al. 1998a). The MDI syndrome does not seem to represent a prodrome state since preliminary 2-year follow-up data suggest that most MDI patients do not progress to more severe chronic psychotic disorders. Similar findings were seen by Lofgren and colleagues (1991) in a prospective follow-up study of 19 severely ill, hospitalized children with many characteristics similar to patients with MDI at ages 6 to 10. At 10- to 20-year follow-ups, the majority of these patients were diagnosed as having severe personality disorders but not schizophrenia or any other Axis I disorder (Lofgren et al. 1991).

Children with MDI and MDD appear to be as numerous as true schizophrenic patients and so are of considerable clinical concern. The possibility that the multidimensionally impaired subjects represent a phenotypic variant of COS, possibly sharing some features related to risk for early onset, remains one of the questions for ongoing research. There have been no treatment studies in patients with MDI or MDD. A double-blind, parallel group comparison of clozapine-olanzapine is ongoing at the National Institute of Mental Health (NIMH) for severely disturbed MDI patients.

Treatment Principles

Children and adolescents with psychotic disorders benefit from a variety of treatments, including medication and psychosocial interventions. The development of a treatment plan requires the consideration of many issues, including current clinical status, cognitive level, developmental stage, and severity of illness. The general principles of the care of children and adolescents with psychotic disorders outlined in this text have been modified from practice guidelines for schizophrenic adults (American Psychiatric Association 1997).

1. Establishing a Therapeutic Alliance

Before starting a drug trial, it is necessary to establish a supportive therapeutic relationship with both the patient and family. At the start of treatment, many patients have difficulty forming trusting relationships and sharing their thoughts, and families might feel stigmatized because their children have a severe mental illness. The formation of an alliance can be facilitated by 1) offering continuity of care with a consistent group of providers, 2) attempting to understand the viewpoint and needs of each patient (e.g., recognizing worries about treatment and maintaining self-esteem and allowing for decreased social contact and/or stimulation in their environment), and 3) paying attention to family members' concerns.

2. Providing Education Regarding Childhood-Onset Schizophrenia and Its Treatments

Open communication among family members, teachers, and caregivers is necessary, because many adolescents with COS often lack insight into the nature of their illness. Open communication should be discussed with both the patient and family early on. Both patients and family members should be made aware of how to recognize changes in mood, behavior, or thought processes that may be indicative of clinical deterioration so that adequate treatment can be provided quickly. This early detection has become especially important because new data suggest that psychotic relapses may have a cumulative effect and accentuate a downhill course (Wyatt et al. 1997).

Almost all families experience considerable distress in dealing with a child or adolescent with schizophrenia or any other psychotic disorder. Regular feedback sessions with families should be offered to discuss the nature of the child's illness, prognosis, and treatment. This process can be started by exploring with the family members their understanding of the cause or causes of their child's illness and explaining to the family that the etiology of schizophrenia is currently unknown. Attention should be given to the psychological factors that impede a patient or family's ability to use information. The process of accepting an illness is lifelong, and with each developmental stage (e.g., graduation from high school or a sibling going off to college) there are new adjustments and realizations. Many parents have appreciated teaching from our staff regarding the symptoms and behaviors associated with their child's disorder, about how to provide the least stressful environment for the child, and problem-solving strategies to deal with disturbing behaviors. Parents often need support to set limits on their child's behavior and to take breaks for themselves. Both individual sessions and group discussion may be helpful. In multiple-family support groups, family members can share their experience of having a psychotic child (e.g., trying to distinguish willful behavior from psychotic symptoms, coping with their own guilt and disappointment, learning how not to personalize their child's rejection or anger, and learning how not to ignore their healthy children).

3. Increasing Understanding of and Adaptation to the Disorder

The disruption associated with a schizophrenic illness in childhood frequently leaves many patients and their families with psychological, academic, and financial issues that require assistance. Health care providers can help patients cope with their environments by improving family relationships and communication skills, teaching personal safety, reviewing educational plans, advocating for special rehabilitative services, accessing appropriate medical care, and securing disability income support when appropriate. Part of this teaching could include identifying for children safe people with whom to share the experience of their illness and how to deal with frightening aspects of their illness.

It is important to give practical advice and support as needed. For example, families may require assistance in dealing with their adolescents' developmentally appropriate needs (e.g., wanting to drive, go to college, live independently, manage sexual feelings, or self-administer medications) and the uncertainty about their children's futures. This latter point has been especially important for approximately one-third of the COS patients in our study who have responded poorly to both typical and atypical neuroleptics.

Pharmacologic Treatments

Therapeutic treatment trials of antipsychotic agents have been a major focus of the Childhood-Onset Schizophrenia Project at the NIMH.

Although there are compelling control trial data to support the use of antipsychotics in adult patients with psychotic disorders, few studies have included pediatric patients (under age 18). Nevertheless, apart from differences in side effects and dosing, treatment efficacy would appear to be similar in both adult and pediatric patients. Because these agents are antipsychotics rather than diagnosis-specific agents, one would infer equality in all affective and nonaffective psychoses. Short-term efficacy has generally been measured by reductions in positive or negative symptoms among treated patients during 4- to 8-week medication trials. An advantage of these studies is that they clearly demonstrate how well a medication can reduce target symptoms; however, less clear is whether symptomatic improvement will lead to improvements in long-term outcome (M. Campbell et al., in press).

In explaining the benefits of drug treatment, it is important to help parents modify expectations for their child while allowing them to maintain hope. All neuroleptic drugs are indicated for the acute and preventative treatment of psychotic episodes, but no curative treatment for psychotic disorders is available. Since the onset of therapeutic effects of neuroleptics may take several weeks, high-dose trials and rapid switching of agents are not helpful (M. Campbell and Cueva 1995a, 1995b).

Pretreatment Screening

A detailed medical workup including 1) measurement of height and weight; 2) neurological examination for tics, stereotypies, extrapyramidal disorders, and tardive dyskinesia; 3) baseline laboratory evaluations (e.g., thyroid function tests, screen for toxic substances, pregnancy test, serum ceruloplasmin, erythrocyte sedimentation rate, antinuclear factor, complete blood count, urinalysis, renal function tests, and liver function tests); 4) magnetic resonance scan of the brain; 5) electroencephalogram; 6) karyotype and molecular fragile X analysis; 7) cerebrospinal fluid analysis (as clinically indicated, especially for acute-onset cases); and 8) genetics examinations are necessary to exclude known medical causes of psychotic disorders in childhood (M. Campbell and Cueva 1995a, 1995b).

Conventional Antipsychotic Medications

Typical neuroleptic drugs (e.g., haloperidol, thiothixene, and loxapine) are acceptable first-line treatments for children with psychotic disorders. The selection of an antipsychotic medication is frequently guided by past response, family history of response, cost, and the patient's tolerance of side effects. Two controlled trials support the use of typical neuroleptics in children and adolescents with schizophrenia (Pool et al. 1976; Spencer et al. 1992).

Spencer et al. (1992) conducted a 10-week, double-blind, placebo-controlled, crossover trial on 16 hospitalized children aged 5.5 to 11.75 years. Diagnosis was made using structured interviews. Haloperidol was found to be clinically and statistically superior to placebo on several measures including the Global Clinical Judgments ratings, reduction of the Brief Psychiatric Rating Scale for Children, total pathology scores, Clinical Global Impressions Scale (CGI) Severity of Illness, CGI Global Improvement, and four Children's Psychiatric Rating Scale (CPRS) items (ideas of reference, persecution, other thinking disorders, and hallucination) (Fish 1985; Guy 1976).

Therapeutic doses of haloperidol ranged from 0.5 to 3.5 mg/day (0.02–0.12 mg/kg/day). The most common untoward effects were excessive sedation and parkinsonian symptoms. Good clinical response to haloperidol was inversely related to duration of illness and positively related to age and level of intellectual functioning (Spencer et al. 1992). These preliminary findings were confirmed at the completion of the study ($N = 24$) (E. Spencer, unpublished data, June 1996). These results are comparable to studies of adult schizophrenic patients, in which the response rate to haloperidol during the first 6 weeks of treatment (as defined by the proportion improving >30% on the Brief Psychiatric Rating Scale [BPRS] [Overall and Gorham 1962] Psychosis Factor) ranges from 20% to 60% (Kane 1996).

Pool and colleagues (1976) conducted a double-blind, placebo-controlled trial comparing haloperidol to loxapine employing a parallel group design in 75 hospitalized adolescents with acute schizophrenia, aged 13 to 18 years. At daily doses ranging from 2 to 16 mg/day (mean 9.8 mg/day) of haloperidol and 10–200 mg/day (mean 87.5 mg/day) of loxapine, there was no statistical difference between drugs and placebo; BPRS ratings reflected significant reduction of symptoms and factors from baseline in all three treatment conditions. However, severely or very severely ill patients tended to show greater improvement on active drugs than on placebo. Untoward effects, mainly parkinsonism and sedation, were common with both haloperidol and loxapine.

Limitations of Conventional Antipsychotic Drugs

The major limitations of conventional antipsychotic drugs in COS patients include inadequate treatment response, lack of efficacy against negative symptoms, galactorrhea, gynecomastia, excessive weight gain, sedation, and neurological side effects (M. Campbell and Cueva 1995a, 1995b; M. Campbell et al., in press; Wolf and Wagner 1993).

In a study of 34 neuroleptic-nonresponsive COS patients, 17 of 34 (50%) were noted to have dyskinesias (9 withdrawal dyskinesia and 8 tardive dyskinesia) at some point during their participation in treatment studies at the NIMH (Kumra et al., in press [b]). In general, for these patients, the dyskinesias were mild to moderate, as rated on the Abnormal Involuntary Movement Scale (Rapoport et al. 1985); involved the muscles of the mouth, tongue, and jaw; improved within 3 months of onset; and were reversible with either drug discontinuation or initiation of clozapine or olanzapine.

COS patients with dyskinesias had significantly poorer premorbid adjustment ($P \leq .02$) and were more likely to have a greater severity of positive symptoms ($P < .01$) (drug free) compared with patients without evidence of dyskinesias (Kumra et al. 1998b). Although it is unclear what pathophysiologic factors might be responsible for increased tardive dyskinesia vulnerability, using the minimum effective dosage of antipsychotic medication is recommended in all cases (Khot et al. 1992). Other neurological side effects including parkinsonian-like symptoms, dystonic reactions, akathisia, and neuroleptic malignant syndrome can also be observed in children treated with typical neuroleptics (M. Campbell and Cueva 1995a, 1995b).

No studies have systematically examined the effects of antipsychotic agents on cognitive functions in schizophrenic children and adolescents. In general, the improvements in attentional impairments and organizational ability outweigh the negative side effects of antipsychotic medications. To allow for early detection of side effects, particularly sedation, the antipsychotic should be administered in divided doses initially (two or three times per day) (M. Campbell and Cueva 1995a, 1995b).

Neuroleptic-Nonresponsive Childhood-Onset Schizophrenia

A substantial proportion of patients with adult-onset schizophrenia fail to respond adequately to antipsychotic medications. Although it is uncertain whether children and adolescents with schizophrenia are actually less responsive to neuroleptic agents (Pool et al. 1976; Spencer et al. 1992), in adult patients earlier age at onset is reported to be a predictor of poor therapeutic response (Meltzer et al. 1997).

Atypical Antipsychotics

All atypical neuroleptics, irrespective of their differing pharmacology, have as an important condition a lesser propensity to produce extrapyramidal side effects and, whether related to this quality or not, enhanced antipsychotic effects. Clozapine, risperidone, and olanzapine are new medications for the treatment of psychotic disorders. These drugs are linked by some characteristic binding profiles to dopamine and serotonin receptors that differentiate these drugs from conventional antipsychotics (Pickar 1995). Both olanzapine and risperidone are acceptable first-line agents for pediatric patients. However, a clozapine trial should be attempted only after two adequate antipsychotic drug trials (Kane 1996).

Risperidone

The key clinical trial supporting the efficacy of risperidone for the reduction of psychotic symptoms was conducted in chronic schizophrenic adults (Marder and Meibach 1994). Armenteros and colleagues (1997) conducted an open pilot study of risperidone in 10 adolescents with acute schizophrenia, aged 11 to 18 years. At daily doses ranging from 4 to 10 mg (mean 6.6 mg), a clinical and statistically significant improvement was seen on the Positive and Negative Syndrome Scale for Schizophrenia (PANSS) (Kay et al. 1987), Brief Psychiatric Rating Scale (Overall and Gorham 1962), and Clinical Global Impression scale. No major adverse reactions were associated with risperidone use. However, extrapyramidal side effects were minimal to mild at low doses but increased at doses above 6 mg/day.

Grcevich and colleagues (1996) conducted a retrospective study of risperidone in 16 children and adolescents with psychotic disorders, aged 9–20 years. At daily doses ranging from 2 to 10 mg (mean 5.9 mg) robust improvements were noted on the Brief Psychiatric Rating Total Score ($P < .0001$) and Clinical Global Impression scale ($P < .0001$). The major adverse effects reported were mild sedation in 5 of 16 (31%) patients and extrapyramidal side effects in 3 of 16 (19%) patients. Other investigators have also described the occurrence of extrapyramidal side effects in children and adolescents receiving low doses of risperidone (Mandoki 1995).

We have described two male patients with psychotic disorders who presented with obesity, liver enzyme abnormalities, and confirmatory evidence of fatty liver (Kumra et al. 1997). Thus, we have recommended that pediatric patients treated with risperidone have baseline liver function tests, careful monitoring of weight, and periodic monitoring of liver function tests during the maintenance phase of therapy. The risk of tardive dyskinesia with risperidone is presently unknown but is probably less than that associated with traditional neuroleptics (Feeney and Klykylo 1996).

Clozapine

Clozapine, the first atypical antipsychotic available in the United States, has not been associated with significant extrapyramidal side effects or dystonia and appears to cause tardive dyskinesia to a much lesser degree than typical neuroleptics or possibly not at all (Kane 1996). The adult data and our own experience clearly show that clozapine is beneficial in a substantial number of patients (30%) who have not improved on multiple trials of typical neuroleptics (Kane 1996; Kumra et al. 1996). Clozapine represents the first drug with convincing data to show that it is superior to any other neuroleptic in the treatment of schizophrenia.

Our center has the most systematic experience in the United States with the use of clozapine in treatment-refractory schizophrenic children and adolescents, having studied 27 children to date in either open or double-blind protocols. The NIMH cohort of neuroleptic-nonresponsive schizophrenic patients is characterized by an equal distribution of males and females, with approximately two-thirds of the patients having developed an insidious onset of their disorder. At the time of referral, many of the patients had already received considerable hospitalization and prior neuroleptic exposure (Kumra et al. 1996). As seen in previous studies (Russell et al. 1989), almost all patients had both positive and negative symptoms of schizophrenia that significantly interfered with functioning (McKenna et al. 1994a).

A double-blind parallel comparison of haloperidol and clozapine in 21 treatment-refractory COS patients (mean age 14.0 years) found clozapine superior to haloperidol for both positive

$(P < .01)$ and negative $(P < .002)$ symptoms and for measures of overall improvement $(P < .04)$ (Kumra et al. 1996). Clozapine doses began at 6.25–25 mg/day, depending on the patient's weight. Doses could be increased every 3–4 days by one to two times the starting dose on an individual basis (Kumra et al. 1996).

The mean dose of clozapine at the sixth week of treatment was 176 ± 149 mg/day (range of 25–525 mg/day). Medical monitoring included weekly complete blood cell counts with differential, liver function tests, an encephalogram, and an electrocardiogram before drug initiation and at week 6 of treatment.

At the completion of a 6-week trial, because of the dramatic improvement in clinical symptomatology and reduction of aggressive outbursts associated with clozapine treatment, many COS patients were able to return to a less restrictive setting. To date, 13 of 21 (62%) patients who participated in this double-blind trial have continued on clozapine for an additional 30 ± 15 months after completion of the study, and continued benefits in overall functioning have been seen at 2-year follow-ups (S. Kumra and L. K. Jacobsen, unpublished data, January 1998).

Unfortunately, as seen in adults, the use of clozapine is associated with serious adverse events such as blood dyscrasias and seizures, and therefore the use of clozapine is reserved for only the most severely ill pediatric patients. In our sample, 7 of 27 (26%) patients have needed to stop otherwise effective clozapine therapy because of serious adverse events: two of these patients have developed neutropenias (absolute neutrophil count <1,500) that recurred with drug rechallenge, three patients developed persistent seizure activity despite anticonvulsant treatment, one patient developed excessive weight gain, and one patient developed a threefold elevation in liver enzymes. In each of these cases, no permanent or long-lasting negative consequences were seen after drug withdrawal.

Olanzapine

Because of the need to find a safer or more effective neuroleptic for children and adolescents, our center has been conducting trials with the second-generation atypical antipsychotic olanzapine in patients with COS. Olanzapine is a thiobenzodiazepine similar to clozapine in mechanism of action, with affinity for $5HT_{2a}$, $5HT_{2c}$, D_1, D_2, D_4, muscarinic (M_1), α_1-adrenergic, and H_1 receptors, with one known exception being that olanzapine lacks the α_2-adrenergic activity of clozapine (Pickar 1995).

A multicenter double-blind, placebo-controlled olanzapine-haloperidol comparison in more than 1,996 adults with schizophrenia and schizoaffective disorder found olanzapine to have a comparable efficacy to haloperidol for positive symptoms and improved efficacy to haloperidol for negative symptoms (Tollefson et al. 1997b). No cases of agranulocytosis or seizures in olanzapine patients were reported.

In a controlled, blinded, long-term study of adult patients with psychotic disorders, the rate of newly emergent tardive dyskinesia was significantly lower in patients receiving olanzapine ($N = 207$, up to 20 mg/day, 237 median days of exposure) than haloperidol ($N = 197$, up to 20 mg/day, 203 median days of exposure) (Tollefson et al. 1997a).

To date, 10 children at the NIMH with schizophrenia have received olanzapine in either open or double-blind trials. In general, olanzapine has been well tolerated by our patients in doses up to 20 mg. Olanzapine doses were initiated at 2.5 mg every other day (<40 kg) or 2.5 mg every day (>40 kg), depending on the child's weight, which could be increased to 2.5 mg/day (<40 kg) or 5 mg/day (>40 kg) on day 3. Thereafter, dosage was adjusted upward (using day 1 of treatment as the start date) by 2.5–5 mg every 5–9 days as determined by the treating physician. The maximum daily dose was 20 mg.

The Clinical Global Impression Scale was used to assess how much patients benefited from an 8-week olanzapine trial compared to their clinical condition upon entry into the study. Of the 10 patients who participated in this trial, 3 were rated much improved, 4 minimally improved, 1 no change, 1 minimally worse, and 1 much worse (Kumra et al., in press [b]). The mean dose of medication at the sixth week of treatment for olanzapine was 17.5 ± 2.3 mg/day (range 12.5–20 mg/day).

The most frequent side effects have included increased appetite, constipation, nausea and vomiting, headache, somnolence, insomnia, difficulty concentrating, sustained tachycardia, increased nervousness, and transient elevation of liver transaminases. The incidence of these minor side effects is comparable to our experience with clozapine in open and double-blind trials. No cases of neutropenia or seizures have occurred with olanzapine. Six of ten (60%) children have continued to take olanzapine (2- to 12-month follow-ups) and in some cases have shown continued improvement after completion of the trial. These data provide preliminary support for the use of olanzapine in treatment-refractory COS.

Maintenance Phase of Treatment

The goals of the maintenance phase are to minimize stress on the patient, provide support to minimize the likelihood of relapse, empower parents to be strong advocates for their children, and integrate the children back into their environments. Based on our own experience and the adult literature (American Psychiatric Association 1997), it is important to leave no gaps in service delivery since many patients are vulnerable to relapse and need support in readjusting in returning to their home communities. In addition, since relapses are part of the expected course of the illness (J. R. Asarnow et al. 1994), provision should be made for respite and wraparound services. With this extra support, patients can often be cared for effectively and safely in a less restrictive setting.

No systematic long-term studies in children and adolescents with psychotic disorders have been conducted to provide guidance for drug treatment. At our center, if a patient has improved with a particular medication regimen, we recommend that he or she continue taking the same medication for the next 6 months, with close monitoring for adverse effects (e.g., tardive dyskinesia, which should be evaluated at every opportunity and results recorded at least every 6 months). After completion of an 8-week treatment trial, many treatment-refractory patients remain symptomatic; thus slow titration of their medication upward to find their optimal dose and/or the addition of adjunctive agents for symptom control (e.g., valproic acid, lithium carbonate, and lorazepam) may be required. After the resolution of an acute psychotic episode, both depressive symptoms and/or persistent negative symptoms may be problematic (S. Kumra, unpublished data, January 1998).

After 6 months to 1 year, stable patients who do not have positive symptoms may be good candidates for dose reduction (Schooler 1991). It is prudent to gradually reduce the medication dose, as long as the patient remains stable, to a level of at least one-fifth of the usual maintenance dose. This practice has been rare in our treatment-refractory sample: only one patient (out of 38) has been able to completely come off medication for a sustained period without adverse effects.

In adult schizophrenic patients it has been suggested that medication discontinuation can be considered for patients with multiple prior episodes who have remained stable for 5 years with no positive symptoms and who are compliant with treatment (Schooler 1991). If discontinuation of antipsychotic medication is attempted, additional precautions—such as gradual dose reduction over several months, more frequent visits, and rapid resumption of medication when schizophrenic symptoms appear—should be instituted.

At times it may be necessary to reevaluate a patient's diagnosis as new information becomes available. It is diagnostically useful to observe children and adolescents with psychotic disorders when they are not taking medication. For seven children and adolescents who were referred to our center with a diagnosis of schizophrenia, at the end of a 4-week drug-free period, we felt that continued neuroleptic treatment was no longer warranted either because the patient was in remission from his or her illness or the original diagnosis of schizophrenia was no longer appropriate (Kumra et al. 1998b).

In addition to medication treatment, specific psychosocial treatment strategies should be introduced as the patient's clinical status stabilizes to improve functional outcome. These interventions include occupational therapy focusing on activities of daily living, social skills training, speech and language therapy, recreational therapy, art therapy, and placement in a specialized school setting.

Knowing a child or adolescent's neuropsychological impairments and assets can be very helpful in planning treatment. For example, it has been documented that certain forms of memory and vigilance deficits in schizophrenic adults may hinder patients' psychosocial adjustment (M. F. Green 1996). The pattern of information processing deficits in COS patients is similar to what has been reported in adult-onset schizophrenia (R. F. Asarnow et al. 1995; Kumra et al. 1998a). Neurocognitive information is most helpful when it is collected during the stable phase of a person's illness.

The Role of Measuring Plasma Concentrations of Drugs

As in adults, pharmacokinetic processes in children and adolescents vary from individual to individual and may be variable within the same individual. Animal studies suggest that children might be more sensitive to the extrapyramidal side effects of neuroleptic drugs (Baldessarini and Teicher 1995; R. Campbell et al. 1988). The half-life of psychotropic drugs in children and adolescents is often unknown. Plasma drug levels can be used to identify patients with low levels who are noncompliant, nonresponders, or rapid metabolizers or to aid in the differential diagnosis of patients with high plasma levels and drug toxicity.

Future Research Directions

Although olanzapine has a more benign side effect profile than clozapine, preliminary data based on a comparison of 23 patients who received 6-week open trials of clozapine and/or olanzapine at our center suggest that clozapine has superior efficacy for both positive and negative symptoms in our group of severely ill children (Kumra et al., in press [b]).

In addition, four patients who were clozapine responsive but who could not continue to take the drug due to serious adverse events received an open trial of olanzapine after having received a double-blind trial of clozapine. For this group, each patient was less symptomatic (as measured by the BPRS total score) at week 6 of treatment while on clozapine compared with olanzapine ($P = .03$) (Kumra et al., in press [b]).

The results of this comparison should be considered preliminary because of the small number of patients studied, lack of randomization, open-label design, and fixed order of drug trials (e.g., most patients received a trial of clozapine first). However, based on these preliminary data, we have started an 8-week double-blind comparison trial of clozapine and olanzapine to directly evaluate the relative safety and efficacy of these treatments. Such a trial might also be able to address the question of whether all seriously ill children with psychotic disorders should receive a clozapine trial.

References

Alaghband-Rad J, McKenna K, Gordon CT, et al: Childhood-onset schizophrenia: the severity of premorbid course. J Am Acad Child Adolesc Psychiatry 34:1273–1283, 1995

American Psychiatric Association: Diagnostic and Statistical Manual of Mental Disorders, 3rd Edition. Washington, DC, American Psychiatric Association, 1980

American Psychiatric Association: Diagnostic and Statistical Manual of Mental Disorders, 3rd Edition, Revised. Washington, DC, American Psychiatric Association, 1987

American Psychiatric Association: Practice guideline for the treatment of patients with schizophrenia. Am J Psychiatry 154(suppl):1–49, 1997

Armenteros JL, Whitaker AH, Welikson M, et al: Risperidone in adolescents with schizophrenia: an open pilot study. J Am Acad Child Adolesc Psychiatry 36:694–700, 1997

Asarnow JR, Tompson MC, Goldstein MJ: Childhood-onset schizophrenia: a followup study. Schizophr Bull 20:599–617, 1994

Asarnow RF, Asamen J, Granholm E, et al: Cognitive/neuropsychological studies of children with a schizophrenic disorder. Schizophr Bull 20:647–669, 1994

Asarnow RF, Brown W, Strandburg R: Children with a schizophrenic disorder: neurobehavioral studies. Eur Arch Psychiatry Clin Neurosci 245:70–79, 1995

Baldessarini R, Teicher M: Dosing of antipsychotic agents in pediatric populations. Journal of Child and Adolescent Psychopharmacology 5:1–4, 1995

Beitchman JH: Childhood schizophrenia: a review and comparison with adult-onset schizophrenia. Psychiatr Clin North Am 8:793–814, 1985

Birmaher B, Baker R, Kapur S, et al: Clozapine for the treatment of adolescents with schizophrenia. J Am Acad Child Adolesc Psychiatry 31:160–164, 1992

Campbell M, Cueva JE: Psychopharmacology in child and adolescent psychiatry: a review of the past seven years, part 1. J Am Acad Child Adolesc Psychiatry 34:1124–1132, 1995a

Campbell M, Cueva JE: Psychopharmacology in child and adolescent psychiatry: a review of the past seven years, part 2. J Am Acad Child Adolesc Psychiatry 34:1262–1272, 1995b

Campbell M, Rapoport JL, Simpson GM: Antipsychotics in children and adolescents. J Am Acad Child Adolesc Psychiatry (in press)

Campbell R, Baldessarini RJ, Teicher MH: Decreasing sensitivity to neuroleptic agents in developing rats: evidence for a pharmacodynamic factor. Psychopharmacology 94:46–51, 1988

Cantor S, Evans J, Pearce J, et al: Childhood schizophrenia: present but not accounted for. Am J Psychiatry 139:758–762, 1982

Caplan R: Thought disorder in childhood. J Am Acad Child Adolesc Psychiatry 33:606–615, 1994

Cohen DJ, Paul R, Volkmar FR: Issues in the classification of pervasive and other developmental disorders: toward DSM-IV. J Am Acad Child Adolesc Psychiatry 25:213–220, 1986

Crow TJ, Done DJ, Sacker A: Childhood precursors of psychosis as clues to its evolutionary origins. Eur Arch Psychiatry Clin Neurosci 245:61–69, 1995

Feeney DJ, Klykylo W: Risperidone and tardive dyskinesia (letter). J Am Acad Child Adolesc Psychiatry 35:1421–1422, 1996

Fish, Children's Psychiatric Rating Scale. Psychopharmacol Bull 21:753–764, 1985

Gordon CT, Frazier JA, McKenna K, et al: Childhood-onset schizophrenia: an NIMH study in progress. Schizophr Bull 20:697–712, 1994

Grcevich SJ, Findling RL, Rowane WA: Risperidone in the treatment of children and adolescents with schizophrenia: a retrospective study. J Child Adolesc Psychopharmacol 6:251–257, 1996

Green MF: What are the functional consequences of neurocognitive deficits of schizophrenia? Am J Psychiatry 153:321–330, 1996

Green WH, Padron-Gayol M, Hardesty AS, et al: Schizophrenia with childhood-onset: a phenomenological study of 38 cases. J Am Acad Child Adolesc Psychiatry 31:968–976, 1992

Greenman DA, Gunderson JG, Cane M, et al: An examination of the borderline diagnosis in children. Am J Psychiatry 143:998–1003, 1986

Guy W: CGI Clinical Global Impressions: ECDEU Assessment Manual, Revised Edition. Rockville, MD, U.S. Department Health, Education and Welfare, 1976, pp 218–222

Hafner HK, Nowotny B: Epidemiology of early-onset schizophrenia. Eur Arch Psychiatry Clin Neurosci 245:80–92, 1995

Hafner HK, Maurer K, Loffler WS, et al: Onset and early course of schizophrenia, in Search for the Causes of Schizophrenia, Vol 3. Edited by Hafner H, Gattaz WF. Berlin, Springer-Verlag, 1995

Hollis C: Child and adolescent (juvenile onset) schizophrenia: a case control study of premorbid developmental impairments. Br J Psychiatry 166:489–495, 1995

Jacobsen LK, Rapoport JL: Childhood onset schizophrenia: implications of clinical and neurobiological research. J Child Psychol Psychiatry (in press)

Jacobsen LK, Walker MC, Edwards JE, et al: Clozapine in the treatment of young adolescents with schizophrenia. J Am Acad Child Adolesc Psychiatry 33:645–650, 1994

Kane JM: Schizophrenia. N Engl J Med 334:34–41, 1996

Kay SR, Fiszbein A, Opler LA: The Positive and Negative Syndrome Scale (PANSS) for schizophrenia. Schizophr Bull 13:261–276, 1987

Khot V, Egan MF, Hyde TM, et al: Neuroleptics and classic tardive dyskinesia, in Drug-Induced Movement Disorders. Edited by Lang AE, Weiner WJ. Mount Kisco, NY, Futura, 1992

Kolvin I: Studies in the childhood psychoses: diagnostic criteria and classification. Br J Psychiatry 118:381–384, 1971

Kowatch RA, Suppes T, Gilfillan SK, et al: Clozapine treatment of children and adolescents with bipolar disorder and schizophrenia: a clinical case series. Journal of Child and Adolescent Psychopharmacology 5:241–253, 1995

Kumra S, Frazier JA, Jacobsen LK: Childhood-onset schizophrenia. Arch Gen Psychiatry 53:1090–1097, 1996

Kumra S, Herion D, Jacobsen LK, et al: Case study: risperidone-induced hepatotoxicity in pediatric patients. J Am Acad Child Adolesc Psychiatry 36:701–705, 1997

Kumra S, Jacobsen LK, Lenane M: Multidimensionally impaired disorder: is it a variant of very early-onset schizophrenia? J Am Acad Child Adolesc Psychiatry 37:91–99, 1998a

Kumra S, Jacobsen LK, Lenane M: The spectrum of neuroleptic-induced movement disorders and extrapyramidal side effects in childhood-onset schizophrenia. J Am Acad Child Adolesc Psychiatry 37:221–227, 1998b

Kumra S, Wiggs E, Krasnewich D, et al: Association of sex chromosome anomalies with childhood-onset psychotic disorders. J Am Acad Child Adolesc Psychiatry (in press [a])

Kumra S, Jacobsen LK, Lenane M: Childhood-onset schizophrenia: an open-label study of olanzapine in adolescents. J Am Acad Child Adolesc Psychiatry (in press [b])

Lofgren DP, Bemporad J, King J, et al: A prospective followup of so-called borderline children. Am J Psychiatry 148:1541–1547, 1991

Mandoki MW: Risperidone treatment of children and adolescents: increased risk of extrapyramidal side effects? Journal of Child and Adolescent Psychopharmacology 5:49–67, 1995

Makowski D, Waternaux C, Lajonchere CM: Thought disorder in adolescent-onset schizophrenia. Schizophr Res 23:147–165, 1997

Marder SR, Meibach RC: Risperidone in the treatment of schizophrenia. Am J Psychiatry 151:825–835, 1994

McClellan J, Werry J: Practice parameters for the assessment and treatment of children and adolescents with schizophrenia. J Am Acad Child Adolesc Psychiatry 33:616–635, 1994

McClellan J, Werry JS, et al: Practice parameters for the assessment and treatment of children and adolescents with schizophrenia. J Am Acad Child Adolesc Psychiatry 36S:177S–193S.

McKenna K, Gordon CT, Lenane M, et al: Looking for childhood-onset schizophrenia: the first 71 cases screened. J Am Acad Child Adolesc Psychiatry 33:636–644, 1994a

McKenna K, Gordon CT, Rapoport JL: Childhood-onset schizophrenia: timely neurobiological research. J Am Acad Child Adolesc Psychiatry 33:771–781, 1994b

Meltzer HY, Rabinowitz J, Lee MA: Age at onset and gender of schizophrenic patients in relation to neuroleptic resistance. Am J Psychiatry 154:475–482, 1997

Overall JE, Gorham DR: The Brief Psychiatric Rating Scale. Psychol Rep 10:799–812, 1962

Parnas J, Schulsinger F, Schulsinger H, et al: Behavioral precursors of schizophrenia spectrum: a prospective study. Arch Gen Psychiatry 39:658–664, 1982

Pickar D: Prospects for pharmacotherapy of schizophrenia. Lancet 345:557–562, 1995

Pool D, Bloom W, Mielke DH, et al: A controlled evaluation of loxitane in seventy-five adolescent schizophrenic patients. Therapeutic Research 19:99–104, 1976

Rapoport J, Connors C, Reatig N: Rating scales and assessment instruments for use in pediatric psychopharmacology research. Psychopharm Bull 21:1077–1080, 1985

Rapoport JL, Giedd J, Kumra S, et al: Childhood onset schizophrenia: progressive ventricular change during adolescence. Arch Gen Psychiatry 54:897–903, 1997

Remschmidt H, Schulz E, Martin M: An open trial of clozapine in thirty-six adolescents with schizophrenia. Journal of Child and Adolescent Psychopharmacology 4:31–41, 1994

Russell AT, Bott L, Sammons C: The phenomenology of schizophrenia occurring in childhood. J Am Acad Child Adolesc Psychiatry 28:399–407, 1989

Schooler NR: Maintenance medication for schizophrenia: strategies for dose reduction. Schizophr Bull 17:311–324, 1991

Shultz SC: Schizophrenia during adolescence (abstract), in Symposium Workbook. Sponsored by the American Psychiatric Association, San Diego, CA, May 17, 1997

Spencer EK, Kafantaris V, Padron-Gayol MV, et al: Haloperidol in schizophrenic children: early findings from a study in progress. Psychopharmacol Bull 28:183–186, 1992

Tollefson GD, Beasley CM, Tamura RN, et al: Blind, controlled, long-term study of the comparative incidence of treatment-emergent tardive dyskinesia with olanzapine or haloperidol. Am J Psychiatry 154:1248–1254, 1997a

Tollefson GD, Beasley CM, Tran PV, et al: Olanzapine versus haloperidol in the treatment of schizophrenia and schizoaffective and schizophreniform disorders: results of an international collaborative trial. Am J Psychiatry 154:457–465, 1997b

Towbin KE, Dykens EM, Pearson GS, et al: Conceptualizing "borderline syndrome of childhood" and "childhood schizophrenia" as a developmental disorder. J Am Acad Child Adolesc Psychiatry 32:775–782, 1993

Van Der Gaag RJ, Buitelaar J, Van Den Ban E: A controlled multivariate chart review of multiple complex developmental disorder. J Am Acad Child Adolesc Psychiatry 34:1096–1106, 1995

Volkmar FR: Childhood and adolescent psychosis: a review of the past 10 years. J Am Acad Child Adolesc Psychiatry 35:843–851, 1996

Walker EF, Savoie T, David D: Neuromotor precursors of schizophrenia. Schizophr Bull 20:441–451, 1994

Watkins JM, Asarnow RF, Tanguay PE: Symptom development in childhood-onset schizophrenia. J Child Psychol Psychiatry 29:865–878, 1988

Werry JS, McClellan JM: Predicting outcome in child and adolescent (early onset) schizophrenia and bipolar disorder. J Am Acad Child Adolesc Psychiatry 31:147–150, 1992

Werry JS, McClellan JM, Chard L: Childhood and adolescent schizophrenic, bipolar, and schizoaffective disorders: a clinical and outcome study. J Am Acad Child Adolesc Psychiatry 30:457–465, 1991

Wolf DV, Wagner KD: Tardive dyskinesia, tardive dystonia, and tardive Tourette's syndrome in children and adolescents. J Child Adolesc Psychopharmacol 3:175–198, 1993

Wyatt RJ, Green MF, Tuma AH: Long-term morbidity associated with delayed treatment of first admission schizophrenic patients: a re-analysis of the Camarillo State Hospital data. Psychol Med 27:261–268, 1997

Yan W, Jacobsen LK, Krasnewich DM: Chromosome 22q11.2 interstitial deletions among childhood-onset schizophrenics and "multidimensionally impaired." Am J Hum Genet (in press)

Chapter 4

Affective Disorders in Children and Adolescents: A Critical Clinically Relevant Review

Stan P. Kutcher, M.D., F.R.C.P.C.

Affective disorders are now recognized as a major psychiatric disorder and mental health concern in children and adolescents (Birmaher et al. 1996a; Goodyear 1995). Current diagnostic practices, utilizing DSM-III-R (American Psychiatric Association 1987) and DSM-IV (American Psychiatric Association 1994) criteria, identify prevalence rates of depressive and bipolar disorders that may occur relatively infrequently in the preschool years, showing a slight rise during the early school years and then a rapid increase in prevalence during adolescence to reach almost to the level of adult prevalence rates by the end of the teenage years. For example, prevalence rates of major depressive disorder (MDD) increase from childhood rates of about 1% through age 6 to 8% by the end of adolescence. The rates of dysthymic disorder are thought to follow a similar pattern, although the evidence for this pattern is less well established (Angold 1987; Birmaher et al. 1996a; K. C. Burke et al. 1990; Fleming et al. 1989; Kutcher et al. 1993).

Manic-depressive disorders pose a more difficult question with regard to establishing the prevalence of the illness since the

I thank Ms. Maureen Brennan, Department of Psychiatry, Dalhousie University, Halifax, Nova Scotia, for administrative and secretarial support.

phenomenology and clinical course of mania in children are currently the matter of some debate (Carlson 1996; Nottelmann 1995; Wozniak et al. 1995). The available literature, however, suggests that bipolar disorder often has its onset in adolescence, and the National Institute of Mental Health (NIMH) epidemiologic catchment area study noted a median age at onset of this illness of 18 years (Regier et al. 1988). The weight of current evidence suggests that the prevalence of bipolar disorder in adolescence approximates 1%, which is not substantially different from that in the adult population (Goodwin and Jamison 1990; Lish et al. 1994; Regier et al. 1988).

Affective disorders (MDD, dysthymia, and bipolar disorder) onsetting in the child and adolescent years are characterized by higher family rates of affective illness than affective disorders onsetting in later life; by high rates of comorbidity, especially with conduct, anxiety, and attention-deficit disorders; by a chronic relapsing course of illness; by impaired short- and long-term social, interpersonal, and vocational functioning; and by increased rates of substance use and a high risk for completed suicide (Duffy et al. 1997; Harrington 1992; Kutcher and Marton 1989; Rodhe et al. 1991). Thus, they constitute an important public health issue, and their optimal treatment is necessary both from an individual or family and a population health perspective.

The pathoetiology of child and adolescent affective illnesses has not been clearly determined to date, but historic models of causality focusing on unidimensional social, family, or psychological factors are clearly inadequate. Although these influences may have pathoetiologic significance, current perspectives suggest a complex relationship among them and central nervous system (CNS) functioning. Recently, interest has been increased in the study of the relationship of neurobiologic variables including neuroendocrine and sleep physiology to the pathophysiology of affective disorders in children and adolescents (Brent et al. 1995; Kutcher and Sokolov 1996).

Currently available treatments for these disturbances run the gamut of social, psychological, family, and psychopharmacologic interventions. Of these, although social, psychological, and family interventions are very commonly utilized by practition-ers, arguably the psychopharmacologic treatments have been the most extensively evaluated in terms of efficacy, tolerability, and general clinical utility (Kutcher 1997b). Usual clinical practice combines pharmacological and psychosocial interventions.

Psychopharmacological treatment of affective disorders in children and adolescents arises from two different conceptual frameworks. The first is that of a percolation model in which psychotropic compounds that have been found useful in the treatment of various affective disorders in adult populations have been studied to determine their potential effectiveness and tolerability in child and adolescent populations (e.g., desipra-mine hydrochloride in adolescent MDD). The second is a more recent development in which neurobiologic models utilizing CNS neurodevelopment as a basis for understanding the control of mood and the onset or pathoetiology of affective illness across the life span has begun to inform research into this area.

Concurrently with this second development has been the fur-ther progress in understanding of CNS systems that are likely to underlie the control of mood and the clinical presentation of dis-turbances in affect. As a result of these advances, models that have previously rather simplistically explained the action of an-tidepressant compounds on the basis of receptor activation are being challenged by a better understanding of the molecular and intracellular mechanisms active in neural systems. These new perspectives provide an opportunity to bridge our understand-ing of the relationships between cellular growth and differenti-ation over the life cycle, the neural control of affect at any given point in the life cycle, and the influence of the external environ-ment on these processes (Duman et al. 1997; Post 1992).

New research in juvenile mood disorders (e.g., studies by McCracken, Poland, and colleagues in animal models) suggests that juvenile and adult animals differ in terms of their serotonin system–mediated adaptive responses and furthermore that very-early-onset stress may compromise the later adaptive ca-pacity of some of these neural systems (McCracken 1997; Poland 1997). These observations using a developmental neural system model are consistent with the earlier hypothesis raised on the basis of clinical research involving primarily noradrenergic antidepressants in adolescents that suggested that, in regards to major depressive disorder at least, juvenile-onset depression may differ substantially from adult-onset depression in the relative involvement of noradrenergic mechanisms and thus in the responsiveness of this disorder to primarily noradrenergic-type antidepressant compounds (Kutcher and Sokolov 1996; Kutcher et al. 1994).

Currently, the field of child and adolescent psychopharmacologic treatment of affective illness is undergoing rapid development, and a number of studies that utilize rigorous double-blind, placebo-controlled conditions and large sample sizes to study the relative efficacy and tolerability of various antidepressant compounds in this population are under way in North America and Europe. The results from these studies were not available at the time of this writing, and thus the review of the literature that follows must be reevaluated once these ongoing efforts have been appropriately analyzed and publicized.

Major Depressive Disorder

A variety of antidepressant compounds including tricyclic antidepressants (TCAs), serotonin specific reuptake inhibitors (SSRIs), monoamine oxidase inhibitors (MAOIs), and a number of novel compounds are currently available for clinical use. These compounds have been systematically evaluated to greater or lesser degrees in the treatment of juvenile MDD (Kutcher 1997a; Rosenberg et al. 1994).

Tricyclic Antidepressants

TCAs have been evaluated in a number of open and double-blind studies in children and adolescents. Overall, the results have not supported the data found in adult studies of these compounds in terms of efficacy and tolerability in the treatment of MDD. In children and adolescents, the weight of currently available evidence suggests that TCAs as a group are indistinguishable in efficacy from placebo and that their use carries significant risk, particularly that of serious cardiac events including sudden death.

Of the available TCAs, imipramine has been the most extensively studied. In open studies of imipramine, Ryan et al. (1986) demonstrated a positive response rate of 44% in a population of 34 study completors with a total daily imipramine dose titrated to a maximum of 5 mg/kg/day. Serum levels of imipramine were not significantly predictive of response. In another evaluation, Ryan and colleagues (1988a) reported on a small number of adolescents who had been treatment resistant to a variety of TCAs who were then augmented with lithium carbonate. However, of this group, only a minority responded significantly. There were no differences in lithium serum levels between responders and nonresponders in this study. Strober and colleagues (1990a) reported response rates of less than one-third in 35 subjects with juvenile-onset MDD and, similarly to Ryan et al. (1988a), could not demonstrate a significant difference in plasma imipramine or desmethylimipramine levels between responders and nonresponders. Puig-Antich and colleagues (1987) found that clinical response to imipramine did not differentiate significantly from placebo in children diagnosed with MDD.

Similarly, Hughes et al. (1990) and Petti and Law (1982) were unable to demonstrate that imipramine was significantly more effective than placebo in well-controlled clinical trials. In contrast, some small clinical trials have reported modest success rates with open-label imipramine treatment (Preskorn et al. 1982; Puig-Antich et al. 1979). Additionally, Preskorn and colleagues (1987) were able to demonstrate a small superiority of imipramine over placebo and suggested that the dexamethasone nonsuppression test might predict differential response.

Desipramine (DMI), an active metabolite of imipramine, has received careful evaluation in juvenile MDD. Boulos and colleagues (1992b) were unable to show significant drug placebo differences in efficacy but noted a high incidence of adverse events associated with the use of this compound. Similarly, Kutcher and colleagues (1994) demonstrated that DMI treatment of adolescents with MMD was not significantly more effective than placebo and that adverse events occurred frequently. These events ranged from minor nonspecific symptoms that caused little disturbance in functioning to significant side effects necessitating withdrawal from study protocol. Klein and Koplewicz (1990) reported similar results in a study of DMI-treated adolescents.

The adverse effects profile of DMI, however, includes cardiovascular complications, especially conduction abnormalities, although the clinical significance of these is unclear (Biederman et al. 1989). Sudden death has been reported in a small number of children treated with DMI (Biederman 1995), and although the pathoetiologic role of DMI in these cases has not been unequivocally established, caution in its clinical use is suggested (Kutcher 1997a; Rosenberg et al. 1994).

Albeit inadequately studied in this population, amitriptyline (AMI) has similarly not shown substantive therapeutic efficacy in the treatment of child and adolescent MDD. Kramer and Feiguine (1981) were not able to demonstrate AMI versus placebo differences in an acute-phase study. Similar results were reported by Kye et al. (1996). The study reported by Kashani and colleagues (1984) suggested a probable therapeutic response to AMI, but its conclusions are difficult to appropriately evaluate due to methodologic difficulties and sample size problems. Nevertheless, given the lack of clearly demonstrated effectiveness of AMI in these studies and the high incidence of adverse events and poor tolerability associated with its multiple receptor activity profile, there is little substantive clinical rationale for the use of this compound in child and adolescent depression.

Nortriptyline, a secondary amine metabolite of AMI, has been extensively investigated, primarily by Geller and colleagues (1986, 1989, 1990). Overall, the data from a variety of carefully conducted scientifically valid studies by this group fail to identify the therapeutic superiority of this compound over placebo in both prepubertal and postpubertal populations. Of particular interest was the report by Geller et al. (1990) in which a nortriptyline-treated MDD group demonstrated a lower response rate than a placebo-treated group.

Taken as a whole, the evidence, albeit based on relatively small sample sizes, does not support the therapeutic efficacy of TCAs in the treatment of MDD in children and adolescents. A variety of possible hypotheses have been advanced to account for these findings, including insufficient studies, small sample sizes, high placebo response rates, heterogeneous populations, high rates of comorbid conditions, neurodevelopmental CNS differences between juveniles and adults, the effects of hormonal factors, pharmacokinetic reasons, and others (Birmaher et al. 1996b). However, the fact remains that given the weight of the currently available scientific evidence, there is little if any support for the routine use of TCAs as a first-line therapy in children and adolescents with MDD. From a practical clinical perspective, the lack of demonstrated efficacy in the available studies, the high incidence of side effects associated with the use of these compounds, the well-known cardiotoxicity of the TCAs (particularly desipramine), and the reported but as yet etiologically unsubstantiated sudden death occurring in children treated with desipramine and imipramine suggest that if TCAs are used in treating MDD in children and adolescents, they should be reserved for special cases in which other treatments have proven to be ineffective or intolerable and that appropriate pretreatment physical evaluation including a comprehensive cardiovascular examination be conducted.

Additionally, the use of TCAs for the treatment of MDD in this population should be carried out only with the full informed consent of the patient and parent, including information about the lack of substantiated treatment efficacy in juvenile MDD, the adverse events profile of the various tricyclic medications and the potential cardiotoxicity of these compounds, and the availability of alternative pharmacotherapies (such as SSRIs), which demonstrate a more benign adverse effect profile.

Monoamine Oxidase Inhibitors

MAOIs were among the first antidepressants shown to be effective in adult populations, and their response rates in this population are similar to that of the cyclic compounds (M. Burke and

Preskorn 1995). In depressed adults, a cluster of symptoms including irritability, rejection sensitivity, hyperphagia, hypersomnia, and mood reactivity identify a subgroup of patients who may show a positive response to MAOIs (McGrath et al. 1992). Thus, MAOIs are relatively well established as an effective treatment for MDD in adults.

The MAOIs can be conveniently classified into two groups, nonreversible and reversible. The nonreversible group (e.g., tranylcypromine and phenelzine) is associated with relatively high rates of treatment-emergent adverse events including a potential for hypertensive crisis. The reversible monoamine oxidase inhibitor (RIMA) moclobemide, at usual therapeutic doses (300–600 mg/day), is considered to demonstrate a significantly lower propensity for these adverse events.

Although the symptom profile for which the MAOIs may show preferential efficacy is well described in juvenile depression, studies of MAOIs in children and adolescents are surprisingly few. Ryan et al. (1988b) have reported an open trial of nonreversible MAOIs in depressed adolescents who were treatment resistant to previous tricyclic pharmacotherapy for MDD. In this group of patients, nonreversible MAOIs were used either as a monotherapy or added in combination to continuing TCA treatment. Dietary complications and adverse events occurred commonly, and less than 50% of the sample was deemed to show both a good therapeutic response and a reasonable compliance with dietary restrictions. Fleming and colleagues (1990) investigated the potential efficacy and tolerability of phenelzine in adolescent depression and were unable to demonstrate therapeutic efficacy in their study. An open trial of tranylcypromine in adolescents with MDD, which was initiated by S. Kutcher (unpublished data, April 1992), was discontinued by the investigator because of an extremely high incidence of hypotensive-type symptomatology including orthostatic dizziness, syncope, exercise-induced fainting, and documented orthostatic hypotension.

The weight of the evidence available at this point certainly does not support the routine use of the nonreversible MAOIs in the treatment of MDD in children and adolescents. Indeed, given the results reported previously and the data from adult samples regarding their side effect profile, their use is known to be compromised by their relatively poor tolerability and the potential for a serious adverse event—a hypertensive crisis. Unfortunately, there has been no substantive published research to my knowledge of the effectiveness and tolerability of moclobemide, the reversible inhibitor of monoamine oxidase in this population. Thus, although it may be of potential benefit and may demonstrate a safer use and better tolerability than the nonreversible MAOIs, given the lack of information regarding moclobemide in this population, its use should not be considered as a first-line treatment option.

Selective Serotonin Reuptake Inhibitors

SSRIs have received the most evaluative attention in psychopharmacologic studies of child and adolescent MDD of all of the available classes of antidepressants. Those currently available in the United States and Canada include sertraline, fluoxetine, paroxetine, and fluvoxamine. Although they are extensively used in the treatment of adult MDD, where they are both effective and relatively well tolerated, relatively little is known about their pharmacokinetic properties in children and adolescents. Compared to TCAs, the SSRIs in adult populations are equally effective yet demonstrate significantly improved tolerability and significantly less cardiotoxicity (Leonard et al. 1997).

A large number of open studies are now available assessing a variety of these compounds, especially fluoxetine and sertraline. When taken as a whole, in these open studies, reported therapeutic response rates have been in the area of 65%–75%. For example, reports by Boulos et al. (1992a), Colle et al. (1994), Jain et al. (1992), Joshi et al. (1989), McConville et al. (1996), Strober (1989), Tierney et al. (1995), and Weiss (1993) are all open, naturalistic trials that have demonstrated this positive therapeutic effect. Additionally, treatment-emergent effects have been generally reported as mild and seem to occur relatively infrequently. On the contrary side, a controlled study by Simeon et al. (1990)

failed to demonstrate the therapeutic efficacy of fluoxetine in juvenile patients with MDD. However, another large, well-conducted placebo-controlled study of fluoxetine in depressed juveniles undertaken by Emslie et al. (in press) has demonstrated the superiority of fluoxetine to placebo along with reasonable tolerability.

In the studies reported earlier, the treatment-emergent adverse events of the SSRIs were generally considered to be mild to moderate and the compounds were, on the whole, fairly well tolerated. There were no reports of significant cardiotoxicity.

However, side effects occur. Overall, the side effects tend to be characterized by gastrointestinal effects rather than the anticholinergic and cardiovascular toxicities of TCAs. Additionally, SSRIs are relatively safe in overdose and are felt to exhibit a wide therapeutic index. CNS side effects such as headaches, extrapyramidal symptoms, tics, self-injurious behavior, possible effects on memory, apathy, and alterations in sleep architecture have been reported (see Leonard et al. 1997 for review). However, the clinical significance of these findings remains unclear, and most of these adverse effects often respond appropriately to decreases in total daily dose.

Additionally, there are sporadic reports in the literature about behavioral activation occurring concurrently with the use of SSRIs including fluoxetine- and sertraline-induced mania or hypomania. Although no well-defined predictive risk factors have been clearly established, a family history of bipolar disorder may be implicated. Behavioral activation as a result of SSRI treatment has been reported by a number of authors including Guile (1996), Riddle et al. (1991), and Tierney et al. (1995). These instances do not seem to meet diagnostic criteria for hypomania and are characterized by symptoms that may be more consistent with an akathisia-type disturbance or that of a mild serotonergic overdrive consistent with toxic serotonin syndrome (Shulman 1995). In most cases, these phenomena can be avoided by clinicians using small initiation doses of the medication and by careful titration of dose increments over longer periods.

Taken as a whole, the weight of the available scientific literature suggests that SSRIs may be of clinical efficacy and may be relatively well tolerated in the treatment of children and adolescents with MDD. However, further investigations are needed using properly controlled studies to confirm these initial impressions. From a clinical perspective, it is not unreasonable for the clinician to preferentially select an SSRI compound for the initial pharmacotherapy of MDD in children and adolescents (Kutcher 1997a, 1997b). As with all pharmacologic treatments, this approach must be taken in a supportive psychotherapeutic setting, utilizing a model of education about the illness and the medications that involves the child and whenever possible the parent or designated caretaker. Informed consent for treatment, the use of standardized and objective or subjective evaluation scales such as the Hamilton Rating Scale for Depression (Hamilton 1960), the Beck Depression Inventory (Beck 1978), or the Children's Depression Inventory should be utilized to monitor symptom change, and the time frame for the initial acute treatment phase should last for 8–12 weeks before making a determination of efficacy.

Additionally, good therapeutic practice would suggest that before initiating treatment with SSRIs, adequate baseline assessments and laboratory evaluation should be performed. This evaluation must always include a thorough diagnostic psychiatric assessment and a review of the medical functional inquiry. Any potential medical problems will need to be followed up with appropriate physical examination and diagnostic testing. However, as a general rule, apart from a pregnancy test in reproductive-age females, no specifically consistent laboratory investigation must be performed before initiation of SSRI therapy. In addition, routine screening cardiograms are probably of little or no value, although a history consistent with cardiovascular difficulties should lead to the appropriate investigations.

Treatment of the MDD acute phase with SSRI compounds should take place over 8–12 weeks. It is now understood that depressive disorders in children and adolescents may take longer to respond to treatment than do adult mood disorders. Thus, an effective acute treatment trial for children and adolescents should include 8–12 weeks at an antidepressant dose within putative therapeutic range. This range is suggested in Table 4–1.

Table 4–1. Suggested total daily doses for SSRI treatment of children and adolescents

Medication	Beginning dose	Initial target dose	Usual maximal dose
Sertraline	25 mg	50 mg	100–200 mg
Fluoxetine	5 mg	20 mg	20–60 mg
Paroxetine	10 mg	20 mg	20–40 mg
Fluvoxamine	50 mg	200 mg	200–300 mg

Note. These doses are guidelines only, taken from the available literature and the author's clinical experience. Doses must be individualized, taking into account side effects and efficacy.

Although the evidence is not available from studies of children and adolescents, data from adult samples suggest that early syndromal relapse is common if pharmacotherapies are discontinued prematurely. Thus, and given the experience of seasoned clinicians, it is reasonable to continue the antidepressant medication at the dose that achieved therapeutic response for 4–6 months following resolution of depressive symptomatology. It can be expected that the associated social, interpersonal, and family disturbances that accompany an episode of MDD may take longer to remit than the symptoms of the illness itself.

A number of options are available for individuals who fail to achieve adequate symptom resolution with the initial treatment. These tactics include optimization of treatment, substitution or augmentation of treatment, or combination treatments (Kutcher 1997a, 1997b). Optimization entails increasing or decreasing the antidepressant dose to try to determine whether a different dose from the initial therapeutic dose will be effective. Dose escalation is the strategy most commonly applied, although the clinician should be aware that dose reduction may sometimes be indicated.

Substitution treatments are well described in the adult literature and entail switching the patient from the initial medication to another antidepressant. Current evidence suggests that patients who do not respond to one of the SSRI medications may often respond to another SSRI medication. Data for children and adolescents regarding this issue are not available. Augmentation strategies include the use of lithium carbonate, thyroid hormone, or stimulants added to the initial SSRI treatment. At this point, there are no reported studies of augmentation strategy in children and adolescents who failed to respond to SSRI treatments, and the two available studies of lithium augmentation of TCAs in adolescents (Ryan et al. 1988a; Strober et al. 1992) are contradictory.

Combination treatments include the addition of an antidepressant from a different class (such as a TCA or MAOI) to an SSRI. Such strategies should be reserved for severely refractory cases and carried out in units specialized in the psychopharmacologic treatment of this population.

Alternative nonpharmacologic intervention for severe refractory depressive disorder, particularly including MDD with psychotic symptomatology, includes electroconvulsive therapy (ECT). However, this topic is outside of the limits of this chapter.

Novel Antidepressants

Recently, a number of new antidepressants have been approved for use in the United States and Canada. These medications include nefazodone, venlafaxine, and, more recently in the United States, mirtazapine. Unfortunately, these compounds have been studied insufficiently to make any decision about their potential efficacy or tolerability in this population. Wilens and colleagues (1997) have reported a series of cases regarding the use of nefazodone in a small sample of children and adolescents with a variety of severe treatment-refractory mood disorders. Their data suggest that nefazodone may be a useful treatment for both the unipolar and depressed bipolar populations, but these results await further detailed study.

Bipolar Disorders

Bipolar disorders in children and adolescents may present somewhat differently from the classic adult form. Available data suggest that, in adolescents at least, bipolar mania is characterized by irritability, rapid cycling, and mixed mood states (Carlson 1996; Steele and Fisman 1997). Depressive episodes often predate the first manic episode, and, once established, bipolar disorder continues in a chronic remitting-relapsing course. Currently, the phenomenology of childhood mania is under debate, with some authors suggesting that childhood mania may be a more chronic and less episodic illness, with the primary affective dimension being that of severe irritability and temper outbursts. This issue remains to be resolved (Carlson 1996; Nottelmann 1995; Steele and Fisman 1997; Wozniak et al. 1995).

A number of thymoleptic medications are available for use in the treatment of bipolar disorder, and most of these have received extensive evaluation in studies of adult patients but significantly fewer assessments in children and adolescents. These compounds include lithium carbonate, divalproex sodium, carbamazepine, and more recently lamotrigine and gabapentin.

In children and adolescents, much less research is available to guide rational psychopharmacologic treatment for bipolar disorder. As reviewed by Alessi and colleagues (1993), lithium carbonate has been used successfully for treating bipolar disorder in both children and adolescents, with blood levels ranging from 0.6 to 1.4 mEq/L being associated with clinical response. Similarly to adults, the available evidence, such as the study by Strober and colleagues (1990b), suggests that prophylaxis of juvenile bipolar disorder is associated with continued lithium use and that relapse is associated with its discontinuation.

Adverse events associated with the use of lithium carbonate in children and adolescents are generally similar to those in adults. However, the effects of lithium on bone growth, thyroid gland development, and kidney function have not been as well studied in the juvenile population. Additionally, available clinical-based evidence suggests that some adverse effects of lithium carbonate may be more pronounced in the adolescent population—particularly weight gain and acne (Kutcher 1997a; Strober et al. 1990b). These features of lithium often make it an unattractive compound for children and adolescents, particularly given their concerns about body image. Additionally, lithium has a narrow therapeutic index, and lithium toxicity constitutes a medical emergency. Signs of lithium neurotoxicity include hyperreflexia, ataxia, dysarthria, delirium, and seizures. In severe cases (serum lithium ≥4 mEq/L), hemodialysis is indicated.

The weight of available evidence for lithium use in this disorder suggests that, in many cases, lithium carbonate may be an effective treatment of bipolar disorder in children and adolescents. However, a substantial number of children and adolescents, indeed probably the majority, may have a form of the illness that is less likely to be responsive to lithium treatment—that is, disorders in which the manic episodes are rapid cycling or mixed states. In these situations, alternative thymoleptics may be more useful (Kutcher 1997a).

The Anticonvulsants

Divalproex sodium has been studied in the treatment of adolescent mania (Papatheodorou and Kutcher 1993; Papatheodorou et al. 1995; West et al. 1994). The evidence from these open studies shows a consistently positive response of the symptoms of acute mania to treatment with divalproex sodium. Additionally, an open-label study by West and colleagues (1995) using an oral loading dose approach in five patients suggested that this method of administering valproate may be equally effective and well tolerated. Serum valproate levels may be related to clinical outcome, and total daily dosings should attempt to establish steady-state serum levels of 50–100 mg/ml. Studies of valproate in the prophylaxis of bipolar disorder are not available for children and adolescents.

The adverse effects of valproate in children and adolescents are similar to those described in adult populations (Kutcher 1997a; Rosenberg et al. 1994). In the acute treatment phase, these side effects include nausea and other types of gastrointestinal distress. Significant weight gain also occurs and may be a rate limiting factor in terms of compliance with long-term prophylactic treatment. Transient increases in hepatic enzymes occur commonly and appear to have little clinical significance. However, fatal hepatotoxicity has been reported in young children treated with valproate and other compounds concurrently, and thus its use is not recommended for preschoolers. Thrombocytopenia may occur with some frequency but rarely requires discontinuation of treatment. Drug-drug interactions may occur with commonly used compounds such as erythromycin, benzodiazepines, or salicylates. Clinicians using valproate should familiarize themselves with the most commonly occurring drug-drug interactions (Kutcher 1997a; Rosenberg et al. 1994).

Another anticonvulsant, carbamazepine, has shown efficacy in adults with acute mania, particularly those who have failed to respond adequately to lithium. However, sufficient data to establish potential utility for children and adolescents are not available for this compound. Carbamazepine use is associated with a number of treatment-emergent adverse events including gastrointestinal distress; neurotoxicity; and the risk for agranulocytosis, aplastic anemia, and exfoliative skin syndromes. Additionally, carbamazepine exhibits numerous drug-drug interactions and is known to induce its own metabolism, thus making this compound perhaps the most difficult of the traditional thymoleptics to use clinically (Kutcher 1997a; Rosenberg et al. 1994).

At this point, insufficient information is available regarding the potential use of the anticonvulsants lamotrigine and gabapentin for bipolar disorder in children and adolescents. Some of the recent evidence suggests that lamotrigine may be effective in adults with bipolar disorder, and this compound has been used for some time in the treatment of epilepsy in childhood. However, its use must currently be considered experimental in treating juvenile bipolar disorder.

The weight of available evidence suggests that a reasonable first-line treatment for bipolar disorder in children and adolescents would be divalproex sodium or, alternately, lithium. This suggestion is consistent with the available literature in studies of adults with bipolar disorder and the available albeit limited literature in juvenile bipolar illness. Although exact dosage parameters have not been determined, the available literature and clinical experience suggest that serum levels in the order of 50–100 µg/ml for valproate and 0.8–1.2 mEq/L for lithium should be targeted.

Baseline investigations before the use of thymoleptics should include a detailed diagnostic assessment and a full medical functional inquiry. Potential physical problems should be followed up with the appropriate diagnostic tests and physical examination.

Baseline laboratory investigations should evaluate parameters that are known to be affected by (or that, if abnormal at baseline, will affect) medication selection. For lithium carbonate, this approach entails the pretreatment measurement of thyroid and renal function, electrocardiogram, and serum electrolytes. With valproate, baseline laboratory screening should include a complete blood count with differential and platelet count. Liver function tests should also be obtained. All females within childbearing years should undergo pregnancy tests, and physicians should keep in mind that these thymoleptics may be associated with cardiac defects (lithium) or with neural tube defects (valproate) during fetal development. Inadequate response to initial thymoleptic treatment should lead the clinician to consider the combining of thymoleptics, particularly lithium, with divalproex sodium. The combination of valproate and carbamazepine should be avoided. Usual daily doses for lithium and valproate in the treatment of acute mania are found in Table 4–2.

The use of antipsychotic medications in treatment-resistant mania is controversial. Some evidence suggests that the new atypical compounds such as clozapine or risperidone may be of value in this population. However, sufficient evidence regarding this indication in children and adolescents is not available in the literature to guide clinical practice. Nevertheless, experienced clinicians report that combining a thymoleptic with an atypical

Table 4–2. Suggested total daily doses for lithium and divalproex sodium in the treatment of acute mania in children and adolescents

Medication	Initial target dose	Suggested serum level
Valproate	1,000–2,500 mg	50–100 mg/ml
Lithium	600–900 mg	0.8–1.2 mEq/L

Note. These doses are guidelines only, taken from the available literature and the author's clinical experience. Doses must be individualized, taking into account side effects and efficacy.

antipsychotic compound such as low-dose (1–4 mg/day) risperidone may be useful in selected cases that are resistant to thymoleptic monotherapy. In these cases, the appropriate strategies for monitoring the extrapyramidal side effects of antipsychotics must be instituted and the potential long-term effects of these compounds such as tardive dyskinesia considered. As always, informed consent from the patient and parent or other caregiver is necessary.

Alternatively, ECT may provide a useful strategy for treatment-resistant bipolar mania. The available literature on this topic suggests that it may be an effective and cost-efficient treatment (Kutcher and Robertson 1995; Papatheodorou and Kutcher 1996). The adverse events of this intervention have not been sufficiently studied in children and adolescents, particularly the long-term cognitive aspects. The details regarding the use of ECT in bipolar disorder of children and adolescents are beyond the scope of this chapter, and the reader is encouraged to consult works by Kutcher and Robertson (1995) and Papatheodorou and Kutcher (1996).

Conclusion

Significant new information has become available over a relatively short period of time to assist the clinician in the selection of psychotropic interventions in the treatment of affective disorders of children and adolescents. However, most of the available studies do not meet type 1 level of evidence (evidence obtained from double-blind, placebo-controlled trials), and judicious clinical practice suggests that in every case, the risks and benefits of treatment must be carefully addressed not only by the clinician but in collaboration with the patient and the patient's family or significant caregiver. Nevertheless, the weight of clinical evidence suggests that for the treatment of affective disorders in children and adolescents, a combination of pharmacologic and psychosocial educational interventions is indicated and, when properly applied and monitored, may be expected to lead to optimal outcomes.

References

Alessi N, Naylor M, Ghaziuddin M, et al: Update on lithium carbonate therapy in children and adolescents. J Am Acad Child Adolesc Psychiatry 33:291–304, 1993

American Psychiatric Association: Diagnostic and Statistical Manual of Mental Disorders, 3rd Edition, Revised. Washington, DC, American Psychiatric Association, 1987

American Psychiatric Association: Diagnostic and Statistical Manual of Mental Disorders, 4th Edition. Washington, DC, American Psychiatric Association, 1994

Angold A: Childhood and adolescent depression, I: epidemiological and etiological aspects. Br J Psychiatry 152:69–78, 1987

Beck AT: Depression Inventory. Philadelphia, PA, Philadelphia Center for Cognitive Therapy, 1978

Biederman J: Sudden death in children treated with a tricyclic antidepressant. J Am Acad Child Adolesc Psychiatry, 30:495–496, 1995

Biederman J, Baldessarini RJ, Wright V: A double-blind placebo controlled study of desipramine in the treatment of ADD, II: serum drug levels and cardiovascular findings. J Am Acad Child Adolesc Psychiatry 28:903–911, 1989

Birmaher B, Ryan N, Williamson D: Depression in children and adolescents: clinical features and pathogenesis, in Mood Disorders Across the Life Span. Edited by Shulman K, Tohen M, Kutcher S. New York, Wiley, 1996a, pp 51–83

Birmaher D, Ryan ND, Williamson DE, et al: Childhood and adolescent depression: a review of the past 10 years, part II. J Am Acad Child Adolesc Psychiatry 35:1575–1583, 1996b

Boulos C, Kutcher S, Gardner D, et al: An open naturalistic trial of fluoxetine in adolescents and young adults with treatment resistant major depression. Journal of Child and Adolescent Psychopharmacology 2:103–111, 1992a

Boulos C, Kutcher S, Marton P, et al: Response to desipramine treatment in adolescent major depression. Psychopharmacol Bull 27:59–65, 1992b

Brent D, Ryan N, Dahl R, et al: Early-onset mood disorder, in Psychopharmacology: The Fourth Generation of Progress. Edited by Bloom FE, Kupfer DJ. New York, Raven, 1995, pp 1631–1642

Burke KC, Burke JD Jr, Regier DA, et al: Age at onset of selected mental disorders in five community populations. Arch Gen Psychiatry 47:511–518, 1990

Burke M, Preskorn SH: Short-term treatment of mood disorders with

---

standard antidepressants, in Psychopharmacology: The Fourth Generation of Progress. Edited by Bloom FE, Kupfer DJ. New York, Raven, 1995, pp 1053–1065

Carlson G: Clinical features and pathogenesis of child and adolescent mania, in Mood Disorders Across the Life Span. Edited by Shulman K, Tohen M, Kutcher S. New York, Wiley, 1996, pp 127–147

Colle LM, Belair JF, DiFero M, et al: Extended open label fluoxetine treatment of adolescents with major depression. Journal of Child and Adolescent Psychopharmacology 4:225–232, 1994

Duffy A, Kutcher S, Alda M, et al: Hypothèsis génétiques et troubles de l'humeur à début précoce, in Les dépressions chez l'enfant et l'adolescent. Edited by Mouren-Simeon MC and Klein RG. Paris, France, Expansion Scientifique Publications, 1997, pp 243–257

Duman RS, Heninger GR, Nesler EJ: A molecular and cellular theory of depression. Arch Gen Psychiatry 54:597–606, 1997

Emslie G, Rush AJ, Weinberg AW: A double-blind, randomized placebo controlled trial of fluoxetine in depressed children and adolescents. Arch Gen Psychiatry 54:1031–1037, 1997

Fleming JE, Offord DR, Boyle MH: Prevalence of childhood and adolescent depression in the community: Ontario Child Health Study. Br J Psychiatry 155:647–654, 1989

Fleming JE, Atley S, Sanford MN, et al: Phenelzine in the treatment of adolescent major depressive disorder: preliminary findings. Poster presentation at the Annual Meeting of the American Academy of Child and Adolescent Psychiatry, San Antonio, TX, October 1990

Geller B, Cooper T, Chestnut E, et al: Preliminary data on the relationship between nortriptyline plasma level and response in depressed children. Am J Psychiatry 143:1283–1286, 1986

Geller B, Cooper T, McCombs H, et al: Double-blind, placebo-controlled study of nortriptyline in depressed children using a "6th plasma level" design. Psychopharmacol Bull 25:101–108, 1989

Geller B, Cooper T, Graham D, et al: Double-blind, placebo-controlled study of nortriptyline in depressed adolescents using a "fixed plasma level" design. Psychopharmacol Bull 26:85–90, 1990

Goodwin FK, Jamison KP: Manic Depressive Illness. New York, Oxford University Press, 1990

Goodyear I (ed): The Depressed Child and Adolescent. Cambridge, MA, Cambridge University Press, 1995

Guile JM: Sertraline induced behavioral activation during the treatment of an adolescent with major depression. Journal of Child and Adolescent Psychopharmacology 2:281–286, 1996

Hamilton M: A rating scale for depression. J Neurol Neurosurg Psychiatry 23:56–62, 1960

Harrington R: Annotation: the natural history and treatment of child and adolescent affective disorders. J Child Psychol Psychiatry 33:1287–1302, 1992

Jain U, Birmaher D, Garcia M, et al: Fluoxetine in children and adolescents with mood disorders: a chart review of efficacy and adverse effects. Journal of Child and Adolescent Psychopharmacology 4:259–261, 1992

Joshi PT, Walkup JT, Cetozzoli JA, et al: The use of fluoxetine in the treatment of major depressive disorder in children and adolescents. Paper presented at the 36th Annual Meeting of the American Academy of Child and Adolescent Psychiatry, New York, October 11–15, 1989

Hughes CW, Preskorn SH, Weller E, et al: The effect of concomitant disorders in childhood depression on predicting treatment response. Psychopharmacol Bull 26:235–238, 1990

Kashani J, Slakeim W, Reid J: Amitriptyline in children with major depressive disorder: a double-blind crossover pilot study. J Am Acad Child Adolesc Psychiatry 23:348–351, 1984

Klein R, Koplewicz H: Desipramine treatment in adolescent depression. Paper presented at the Child Depression Consortium Meeting, Pittsburgh, PA, September 1990

Kramer A, Feiguine R: Clinical effects of amitriptyline in adolescent depression. Journal of the American Academy of Child Psychiatry 20:636–644, 1981

Kutcher S: Child and Adolescent Psychopharmacology. Philadelphia, PA, WB Saunders, 1997a

Kutcher S: Practitioner review: the pharmacotherapy of adolescent depression. J Child Psychol Psychiatry 38/7:755–767, 1997b

Kutcher S, Marton P: Parameters of adolescent depression: a review. Psychiatr Clin North Am 12:895–918, 1989

Kutcher SP, Robertson H: Electroconvulsive treatment in acute adolescent mania. Journal of Child and Adolescent Psychopharmacology 5:167–175, 1995

Kutcher S, Sokolov S: Adolescent depression: neuroendocrine aspects, in The Depressed Child and Adolescent. Edited by Goodyear IM. Cambridge, MA, Cambridge University Press, 1996, pp 195–224

Kutcher S, Marton P, Boulos C: Adolescent depression: update and review, in Depression and the Social Environment: Research and Intervention With Neglected Populations, Vol 3. Edited by Cappeliez P, Flynn R. Montreal, McGill-Queen's University Press, 1993, pp 77–92

Kutcher S, Boulos C, Ward B, et al: Response to desipramine treatment in adolescent depression: a fixed dose, placebo controlled trial. J Am Acad Child Adolesc Psychiatry 33:686–694, 1994

Kye CH, Waterman GS, Ryan ND: A randomized, controlled trial of amitriptyline in the acute treatment of adolescent major depression. J Am Acad Child Adolesc Psychiatry 35:1139–1144, 1996

Leonard HL, March J, Rickler KC, et al: Pharmacology of the selective serotonin reuptake inhibitors in children and adolescents. J Am Acad Child Adolesc Psychiatry 36:725–736, 1997

Lish JD, Dine MS, Whybrow PC, et al: The National Depressive and Manic-Depressive Association (DMDA) survey of bi-polar members. J Affective Disord 31:281–294, 1994

McConville BJ, Minnery KL, Sorter MT, et al: An open study of the effects of sertraline on adolescent major depression. Journal of Child and Adolescent Psychopharmacology 6:41–51, 1996

McCracken J: Age effects on 5-HT responses after antidepressants. Annual Meeting of the American Academy of Child and Adolescent Psychiatry and the Canadian Academy of Child Psychiatry, Toronto, Canada, October 1997

McGrath P, Stewart J, Harrison W: Predictive value of symptoms of a typical depression for differential drug outcome. J Clin Psychopharmacol 12:197–202, 1992

Nottelmann ED: Special section: bipolar affective disorder. J Am Acad Child Adolesc Psychiatry 34:705–763, 1995

Papatheodorou G, Kutcher S: Divalproex sodium treatment in late adolescent and young adult acute mania. Psychopharmacol Bull 29:213–219, 1993

Papatheodorou G, Kutcher S: Treatment of bipolar disorder in adolescents, in Mood Disorders Across the Life Span. Edited by Shulman K, Tohen M, Kutcher S. New York, Wiley, 1996, pp 101–126

Papatheodorou G, Kutcher S, Katic M, et al: The efficacy and safety of divalproex sodium in the treatment of acute mania in adolescents and young adults: an open clinical trial. J Clin Psychopharmacol 15:110–116, 1995

Petti T, Law W: Imipramine treatment of depressed children: a double-blind pilot study. J Clin Psychopharmacol 2:107–110, 1982

Poland R: Long-term consequences of prenatal stress on 5-HT system. Annual Meeting of the American Academy of Child and Adolescent Psychiatry and the Canadian Academy of Child Psychiatry, Toronto, Canada, October 1997

Post RM: Transduction of psychosocial stress into the neurobiology of recurrent affective disorder. Am J Psychiatry 149:999–1010, 1992

Preskorn SH, Weller EB, Weller RA: Depression in children: relationship between plasma imipramine levels and response. J Clin Psychiatry 43:450–453, 1982

Preskorn SH, Weller EB, Hughes CW, et al: Depression in prepubertal children: dexamethasone non-suppression predicts differential response in imipramine versus placebo. Psychopharmacol Bull 23:128–133, 1987

Puig-Antich J, Perel J, Lupatkin W: Plasma levels of imipramine (IMI) and desmethylimipramine (DMI) and clinical response to prepubertal major depressive disorder: a preliminary report. Journal of the American Academy of Child Psychiatry 18:616–627, 1979

Puig-Antich J, Perel JM, Lupatkin W, et al: Imipramine in prepubertal major depressive disorder. Arch Gen Psychiatry 44:81–89, 1987

Regier DA, Boyd JH, Rae DS, et al: One-month prevalence of mental disorders in the United States: based on five epidemiologic catchment area sites. Arch Gen Psychiatry 45:977–986, 1988

Riddle MA, King RA, Hardin MT, et al: Behavioral side effects of fluoxetine in children and adolescents. Journal of Child and Adolescent Psychopharmacology 1:193–198, 1991

Rodhe P, Lewinsohn PM, Seeley JR: Comorbidity of unipolar depression, II: comorbidity with other mental disorders in adolescents and adults. J Abnorm Psychol 100:214–222, 1991

Rosenberg DR, Holttum J, Gershon S: Textbook of Pharmacotherapy for Child and Adolescent Psychiatric Disorders. New York, Brunner/Mazel, 1994

Ryan ND, Puig-Antich J, Cooper T, et al: Imipramine in adolescent major depression: plasma level and clinical response. Acta Psychiatr Scand 73:275–288, 1986

Ryan ND, Meyer V, Pachille S, et al: Lithium anti-depressant augmentation in TCA-refractory depression in adolescents. J Am Acad Child Adolesc Psychiatry 27:371–376, 1988a

Ryan ND, Puig-Antich J, Rabinovich H: MAOIs in adolescent major depressive disorder and responsive to tricyclic antidepressants. J Am Acad Child Adolesc Psychiatry 27:755–758, 1988b

Shulman R: The serotonin syndrome: a tabular guide. Canadian Journal of Clinical Pharmacology 2:139–144, 1995

Simeon JG, Ferguson HB, DiNicola VF, et al: Adolescent depression: a placebo controlled fluoxetine treatment study and follow up. Prog Neuropsychopharmacol Biol Psychiatry 14:791–795, 1990

Steele P, Fisman S: Bipolar disorder in children and adolescents: current challenges. Can J Psychiatry 42:632–636, 1997

Strober M: Effective imipramine, lithium, and fluoxetine in the treatment of adolescent major depression. NIMH New Clinical Drug Evaluation Unit (NCDEU) Annual Meeting, Key Biscayne, FL, June 4–6, 1989

Strober M, Freeman R, Rigalis J: The pharmacotherapy of depressive illness in adolescents, I: an open label trial of imipramine. Psychopharmacol Bull 26:80–84, 1990a

Strober M, Morrell W, Lampert C, et al: Relapse following discontinuation of lithium maintenance therapy in adolescents with bipolar I illness: a naturalistic study. Am J Psychiatry 147:457–461, 1990b

Strober M, Freeman R, Rigali J, et al: The pharmacotherapy of depressive illness in adolescents, II: effects of lithium augmentation in nonresponders to imipramine. J Am Acad Child Adolesc Psychiatry 31:16–20, 1992

Tierney E, Joshi PT, Linas JF, et al: Sertraline for major depression in children and adolescents: preliminary clinical experience. Journal of Child and Adolescent Psychopharmacology 6:13–27, 1995

Weiss M: Fluoxetine treatment of adolescent depression. Child Depression Consortium Meeting, Toronto, Canada, September 1993

West SA, Keck PE, McElroy SL, et al: Open trial of valproate in the treatment of adolescent mania. Journal of Child and Adolescent Psychopharmacology 4:263–267, 1994

West SA, Keck PE, McElroy SL: Oral loading the doses in the valproate treatment of adolescents with mixed bipolar disorder. Journal of Child and Adolescent Psychopharmacology 5:225–228, 1995

Wilens T, Spencer T, Biederman J, et al: Case study: nefazodone for juvenile mood disorders. J Am Acad Child Adolesc Psychiatry 36:481–485, 1997

Wozniak J, Biederman J, Kiely K, et al: Mania-like symptoms suggestive of childhood onset bipolar disorder in clinically referred children. J Am Acad Child Adolesc Psychiatry 34:867–876, 1995

Chapter 5

Anxiety Disorders

Daniel S. Pine, M.D., and Joseph Grun, B.S.

The term *anxiety* refers to the presence of fear or apprehension that is out of proportion to the context of the life situation. Hence, extreme fear or apprehension is considered an indicator of an anxiety disorder if it is developmentally inappropriate (i.e., fear of separating from a parent in a 10-year-old child) or if it is inappropriate to an individual's life circumstances (i.e., worries that one's family will starve despite financial security) (Barlow 1988; Marks 1988).

In the field of child psychiatry, research on the etiology and treatment of anxiety disorders has traditionally lagged behind research in the areas of disruptive behavior or depressive disorders. As a result, there are relatively fewer data on pharmacological approaches to childhood anxiety disorders than to these other families of disorders. In this context of limited information, the pharmacological approach to childhood anxiety disorders draws heavily on a wealth of literature in the treatment of adult anxiety disorders. In this chapter we therefore review pharmacological approaches to childhood anxiety disorders with extensive reference to approaches among adults.

We cover four specific topics in this chapter. First, clinical descriptions of each anxiety disorder, as currently outlined in DSM-IV (American Psychiatric Association 1994), are provided. Second, given the emphasis on data for adult anxiety disorders in the treatment of children, literature that suggests a close connection between child and adult anxiety disorders is summarized. Third, existing data from pharmacological studies in childhood anxiety disorders are reviewed, with a particular emphasis

This work was supported by NIMH Center Grant MH-43878 to the Center to Study Youth Anxiety, Suicide, and Depression and a Scientist Development Award for Clinicians from NIMH to Dr. Pine (K20-MH01391).

on data from randomized controlled trials conducted since the refinement of the psychiatric nosological system in 1980, with the publication of DSM-III (American Psychiatric Association 1980). Fourth, clinical guidelines for the use of various medications in children with anxiety disorders are provided.

Clinical Features of Childhood Anxiety Disorders

Although anxiety disorders were broadly conceptualized in the early twentieth century, the last 30 years of research among adults has led to narrower definitions of each disorder. This refinement in diagnosis was partially stimulated by pharmacological distinctions among the various adult anxiety disorders. At least among adults, consensus has emerged on the view of anxiety disorders as a family of related but distinct mental disorders.

For both children and adults, DSM-IV considers a group of nine conditions to be primary anxiety disorders: panic disorder with and without agoraphobia, agoraphobia without panic disorder, specific phobia, social phobia, obsessive-compulsive disorder, posttraumatic stress disorder (PTSD), acute stress disorder, and generalized anxiety disorder. A tenth anxiety disorder, separation anxiety disorder, is a specific disorder of children. Although selective mutism, another disorder, is not considered an anxiety disorder in DSM-IV, this condition is frequently complicated by social phobia.

In this chapter we discuss the treatment of 5 of these 11 disorders: panic disorder, with and without agoraphobia; separation anxiety disorder; social phobia; selective mutism; and generalized anxiety disorder. Given the close relationship between selective mutism and social phobia, these disorders are discussed together.

Separation Anxiety Disorder

Separation anxiety disorder is probably the most common impairing anxiety disorder seen in children and adolescents, with epidemiological studies suggesting a prevalence of between 5% and 10% (Costello and Angold 1995). The key feature of this disorder is recurrent fear of separation from the home or from loved ones. As described in DSM-IV, this fear is associated with worries about harm befalling the child or attachment figure, marked distress at times of separation, refusal to separate, nightmares or trouble sleeping, and frequent physical complaints at times of separation.

Children with separation anxiety disorder can present in many clinical scenarios. Some of the most common presentations involve a child's refusal to comply with necessary routines. For example, children who refuse to attend school are often brought for treatment at the insistence of school authorities, or parents might request an evaluation when a child's refusal to stay with a baby-sitter disrupts other routines. Although children with separation anxiety disorder usually acknowledge their internal strife related to anxiety, it is unusual for a referral to start with the request from a child.

Separation anxiety disorder must be differentiated from the normal, developmentally appropriate stage of separation anxiety, which occurs at a much earlier stage, in the first few years of life (R. G. Klein 1995b; Marks 1988). By the time children reach school age, extreme separation fears are almost always indicative of an underlying problem, though this problem is not always separation anxiety disorder. For example, children who have been traumatized, children with depressive disorders, and children with pervasive developmental disorders often present with separation fears. Each of these conditions, however, can be readily distinguished from separation anxiety disorder by their associated features.

Panic Disorder With and Without Agoraphobia

Panic attacks are characterized as episodes of abrupt, intense fear, accompanied by at least four autonomic or cognitive symptoms (listed in Pollack and Smoller 1995). The panic attack must develop rapidly, with anxiety that escalates to a crescendo within minutes and ends abruptly, typically lasting less than 30 minutes. DSM-IV recognizes three types of panic attacks, but only the spontaneous panic attack, which occurs without cue or warning, is an indicator of panic disorder. Panic disorder requires the presence of at least two spontaneous panic attacks, at least one of which is associated with concern about additional attacks, worry about attacks, or changes in behavior that last at least 1 month.

Although panic disorder is a rare condition in adolescents and is extremely rare before puberty, panic attacks are relatively common in children and adolescents. The typical attacks seen in childhood, however, are usually situationally triggered rather than spontaneous. For example, children with separation anxiety disorder often develop panic attacks when separated, while children with phobias often exhibit panic attacks when confronted with a feared object or social scenario. Such panic attacks should not be confused with the spontaneous attacks of panic disorder.

Patients with panic disorder present with a number of co-morbid conditions, but there has been considerable interest in the relationship between panic disorder and agoraphobia, which refers to fear or anxiety related to places from which escape might be difficult (Magee et al. 1996). There remains considerable controversy on the distinctness of agoraphobia as a condition that is separate from panic disorder, a controversy centering on the frequency with which patients develop agoraphobia in the absence of panic disorder or panic attacks (Eaton et al. 1991; R. G. Klein 1995a; Marks 1988). Although DSM-IV suggests that such patients do exist, virtually all patients with agoraphobia who seek treatment suffer from panic attacks. In children and adolescents, it is far more common to encounter patients with separation anxiety disorder who refuse to go to various places because of their fears of separation than to encounter patients with panic disorder complicated by agoraphobia.

Social Phobia and Selective Mutism

The term *phobia* refers to an excessive fear of a specific object, circumstance, or situation (Magee et al. 1996). Phobias are classified based on the nature of the feared object or situation, and DSM-IV recognizes three distinct classes of phobia: agoraphobia, specific phobia, and social phobia. Social phobia is characterized by intense anxiety, even to the point of a panic attack, upon exposure to situations in which an individual is scrutinized and might be embarrassed. It can involve specific fears about performing certain activities, such as writing, eating, or speaking in front of others, or a vague, nonspecific general fear of embarrassing oneself. Individuals with social phobia who fear most situations are considered to suffer from generalized social phobia.

The clinician should recognize that many children and adolescents exhibit at least some degree of social anxiety or self-consciousness, yet few of them meet criteria for social phobia. Anxiety about social or performance situations must either interfere with a child's ability to function or cause a great deal of internal strife for such social anxiety to be considered an indicator of social phobia (Ianlongo et al. 1995). Selective mutism is a disorder that usually presents in childhood and is considered to be closely related to social phobia. Selective mutism is characterized by a child's failure or refusal to speak in social situations. It should be noted that children with selective mutism do not always present with social phobia, and the clinician should elicit other symptoms of social anxiety before concluding as such. In suggestive cases, parents or teachers can virtually always provide other clear signs of extreme social anxiety.

As with other anxiety disorders, social phobia frequently co-occurs with other mood and anxiety disorders (Gurley et al. 1996; Magee et al. 1996). Among adults, the association of social phobia with both panic disorder and major depression has received considerable attention in recently published literature. In children, the association with generalized anxiety disorder appears most prominent. In fact, the strong overlap between social phobia and overanxious disorder, a DSM-III and DSM-III-R (American Psychiatric Association 1987) condition that was subsumed under generalized anxiety disorder in DSM-IV, contributed to the reconceptualization of overanxious disorder in DSM-IV.

Generalized Anxiety Disorder

Generalized anxiety disorder involves frequent, persistent worry and anxiety out of proportion to the circumstances that are the focus of the worry (Schweizer 1995). For example, while children often worry about examinations, a child who persistently worries about failure despite consistently outstanding grades shows the pattern of worry that is typical of generalized anxiety disorder. Similarly, even adolescents with no psychiatric disorder often worry about their popularity, but an adolescent who cannot stop worrying that he or she is not popular enough shows signs that are indicative of generalized anxiety disorder. Children with generalized anxiety disorder may not acknowledge the excessive nature of their worry but must be bothered by their degree of worry. This pattern must occur more days than not for at least 6 months. The child must find it difficult to control this worry. Although a child may or may not acknowledge this difficulty, in children with long-standing worries, historical information from a parental informant virtually always indicates signs of uncontrollable worry. The child must report at least one of six somatic or cognitive symptoms, though adults must report three such symptoms. These symptoms include feelings of restlessness, fatigue, muscle tension, and insomnia. Again, children with chronic worries virtually always exhibit at least one such symptom. Finally, worry is a ubiquitous feature of many anxiety disorders: patients with panic disorder often worry about panic attacks, patients with social phobia worry about social encounters, and patients with obsessive-compulsive disorder worry about their obsessions. The worries in generalized anxiety disorder must be beyond the worries characteristic of these other anxiety disorders.

Relationships Between Childhood and Adult Anxiety

Given that the pharmacological approach to childhood anxiety disorders draws heavily on research with adults, it is important to note the growing research base that links childhood and adult anxiety disorders. As reviewed briefly in the current chapter, this research base essentially draws on three types of studies: family-genetic studies, biological studies, and longitudinal research.

Family-Genetic Studies

Family studies examine the distribution of psychiatric diagnoses among relatives with and without various types of disorders (Fyer et al. 1995). Family studies among adults with various types of psychiatric disorders point to the importance of continued research on children, since these studies find that childhood-onset disorders tend to be more familial than disorders with an onset later in life. While the most extensive literature considers this issue in depression, recent work with panic disorder suggests that child or adolescent onset of this illness, as with major depression, predicts increased familial loading of the disorder (Goldstein et al. 1997; Silove et al. 1995). These findings, however, are limited by the fact that the illness age at onset is usually estimated from retrospective reports of chronically ill adults.

Importantly, as with these studies among adults, findings from a series of research studies directly with children leave little doubt that there are relatively strong relationships between anxiety disorders in children and their parents. For example, children of parents with anxiety disorders are known to face a two- to fourfold increased risk for childhood anxiety disorders (Beidel and Turner 1997; Warner et al. 1995), while parents of children with anxiety disorders are known to face a two- to fourfold increased risk for anxiety disorders (Last et al. 1991).

One open question in research on the association of anxiety disorders in children and their parents pertains to the degree of specificity in familial associations. For example, across family studies, associations among panic disorder, separation anxiety disorder, and overanxious disorder all have been noted, as well as associations between major depression and generalized anxiety disorder. Moreover, the risk for anxiety disorders in children of parents with major depression appears as strong as the risk for depression in such children (Beidel and Turner 1997; Breslau et al. 1987; Warner et al. 1995). As noted earlier, the risk for anxiety disorders in children of parents with anxiety disorders is also quite strong. Although the mechanisms accounting for such family patterns remain poorly understood, possible contributing factors include comorbidity in parents or children and shared risk factors among disorders.

Although this research clearly points to the familial nature of childhood anxiety disorders, these findings leave open the question as to whether genetic or environmental factors account for concordant familial patterns of illness. On the one hand, twin studies in adults and children suggest moderate genetic effects on anxiety symptoms (Thapar and McGuffin 1996). On the other hand, twin studies also suggest moderate to large environmental effects, particularly for nonshared environmental variables (Kendler et al. 1995; Pike et al. 1996).

Biological Studies

A series of studies finds that the biology of childhood anxiety disorders bears similarities to the biology of adult anxiety disorders. Various anxiety disorders of adults, including generalized anxiety and panic disorders, are associated with abnormalities in endocrinological systems that mediate growth, including the growth hormone and hypothalamic-pituitary-adrenal systems. Consistent with such research among adults, longitudinal research with adolescents shows that adolescent girls with anxiety disorders grow up to be nearly 2 inches shorter than their age-mates, despite having normal growth from childhood to early adolescence (Pine et al. 1996).

Beyond research on the neuroendocrinology of adult anxiety disorders, there has also been particular interest in the physiological correlates of adult anxiety disorders observable in the respiratory system. Some adult anxiety disorders, particularly panic disorder, are associated with abnormalities in respiratory physiology, possibly related to abnormalities in the neural control of breathing (D. F. Klein 1993). For example, panic disorder among adults is associated with prominent respiratory symptoms, and adult respiratory illnesses are frequently associated with anxiety disorders, particularly panic disorder. Moreover, there is evidence of increased sensitivity to suffocation cues among adults with panic disorder, manifested as increased dyspnea and abnormal respiratory responses to carbon dioxide, lactate, and other respiratory stimulants. A number of theories attempt to account for these well-replicated findings. For example, it has been suggested that panic disorder results from a hypersensitive suffocation alarm or from abnormalities in various neural systems involved in respiratory control. Other theories emphasize cognitive aspects of suffocating stimuli. Across theories, however, there is a strong, consistent emphasis on the role of respiratory factors in panic-related disorders.

Recent research has begun to extend these findings from adults to children with anxiety disorders. For example, consistent with the data among adults, a series of studies among children with asthma and other chronic illnesses note a strong, specific association between childhood anxiety and respiratory illnesses with prominent smothering symptoms (Mrazek 1992; Pine et al. 1994; Wambalt et al. 1996). Moreover, recent work suggests that some children with anxiety disorders, particularly with separation anxiety disorder, exhibit enhanced sensitivity to CO_2, much like many adults with panic disorder (Pine et al., in press). Ongoing studies are continuing to extend these findings across age and diagnostic groups.

Longitudinal Studies

A large proportion of adults with various impairing disorders, including major depression, panic disorder, and social phobia, report a childhood history of problems with anxiety. These data must be interpreted with caution, given the possibility of selective recall for negative childhood feelings among adults with psychiatric disorders. Prospective studies examining the outcome of children with anxiety disorders over time are needed to critically appraise the suggestion from these studies that childhood anxiety can presage long-term impairment.

Until recently, there have been relatively few prospective data on the outcome of children with anxiety disorders beyond a few long-term studies of obsessive-compulsive disorder against which to view retrospective studies among adults. The few long-term follow-up studies of childhood anxiety disorders, besides obsessive-compulsive disorder, suggest that most children and adolescents with an anxiety disorder fare well over time (Pine et al. 1998; Last et al. 1996). Nevertheless, there are also data to suggest that the majority of late-adolescent or early-adulthood anxiety and depressive disorders are preceded by childhood anxiety disorders. Taken together, these data suggest that while childhood anxiety disorders often remit, a significant proportion of early-adult anxiety disorders arise during childhood. These findings emphasize the importance of identifying factors that distinguish children with transient as opposed to persistent anxiety.

Beyond the issue of persistence in childhood anxiety disorders, questions remain on the specific relationships among the disorders over time. Some evidence suggests both specificity and nonspecificity in the course of the individual anxiety disorders. For example, some data suggest that childhood or adolescent social phobia exhibits a relatively specific course, predicting primarily social phobia in adulthood but not other disorders (Pine et al. 1998). Similarly, both childhood or adolescent panic attacks and separation anxiety disorder have been specifically tied to later-life panic disorder (R. G. Klein 1995a). Other relationships among other disorders, in contrast, appear less specific. Very strong associations exist between major depressive disorder and generalized anxiety disorder during both childhood and adulthood. These associations are consistent with the suggestions from twin studies that major depression and generalized anxiety disorder may share common genes but become distinct disorders through environmental effects during development (Kendler et al. 1995).

Efficacy of Medications in Childhood Anxiety Disorders

A considerable discrepancy remains between the amount of research on the treatment of childhood anxiety disorders and the prevalence of the disorders. As a group, childhood anxiety disorders are probably the most common class of psychiatric disorder affecting children, with a prevalence rate in the 10%–20% range (Costello and Angold 1995). Despite this high prevalence, only a handful of controlled medication trials have been conducted.

The current review emphasizes findings from psychopharmacologic research on the treatment of childhood anxiety disorders based on the randomized, controlled design. Although data from open trials provide valuable information on the tolerability of potential treatments and the feasibility of a controlled trial, such data are of limited use in making judgments about efficacy. Childhood anxiety disorders tend to exhibit a waxing and waning course (Pine et al. 1998). Moreover, nonpharmacological interventions are known to reduce symptoms dramatically for some children with anxiety disorders (Kendall 1994). As a result, one can attribute improvement in symptoms to a medication only when it is used in a randomized, controlled fashion.

For the anxiety disorders considered in this chapter, there have been fewer than 10 randomized, controlled psychopharmacology trials (see Table 5–1). Such randomized, controlled trials have been conducted with three classes of medication: tricyclic antidepressants (TCAs), benzodiazepines, and serotonin reuptake inhibitors. The data from the trials for each class of medication are briefly reviewed.

For the TCAs, there have been four trials in total, one that used clomipramine in the treatment of school refusal, which was felt to be a form of separation anxiety disorder (Berney et al. 1981), and three that used imipramine for the treatment of separation anxiety disorder, usually complicated by school refusal (Bernstein et al. 1990; Gittelman-Klein and Klein 1971; R. G. Klein et al. 1992). Only one of the trials produced clearly positive results

Table 5–1. Randomized, controlled psychopharmacology trials for anxiety disorders in children and adolescents

Source of study	Class of active medications	Superiority over placebo?	Comments
Tricyclic antidepressants			
Berney et al. (1981)	Clomipramine vs. placebo	No	While this study did not provide evidence of clomipramine's benefit, it has been criticized on the grounds that it employed a relatively low dose of clomipramine (to 75 mg maximum).
Bernstein et al. (1990)	Imipramine and alprazolam vs. placebo	No	This study found no consistent differences among study medications. However, the study had limited power because of small sample sizes in three study groups and produced some suggestive evidence supporting the efficacy of the active compounds.
Gittelman-Klein and Klein (1971)	Imipramine vs. placebo	Yes	This study, in a group of children with school refusers, treated before the DSM-III categorization of separation anxiety disorder, remains the only report clearly showing the efficacy of a medication for childhood anxiety besides obsessive-compulsive disorder.
Klein et al. (1992)	Imipramine vs. placebo	No	This study in children with separation anxiety disorder failed to provide any evidence supporting the earlier results from Gittelman-Klein and Klein (1971). This failure occurred despite an identical design as in the earlier study.

Benzodiazepines			
Bernstein et al. (1990)	Imipramine and alprazolam vs. placebo	No	As noted above, interpretation of the data from this study is limited by the small sample size.
Graae et al. (1994)	Clonazepam vs. placebo	No	This study examined the response of 11 subjects with overanxious and other disorders in a crossover design. Although patients generally improved, the improvements were not better than those seen with placebo, and children exhibited signs of disinhibition.
Simeon et al. (1992)	Alprazolam vs. placebo	No	This small study provided some limited evidence of benefit in overanxious and avoidant disorders, though overall improvement did not differ during active treatment.
Kutcher et al. (1992)	Clonazepam vs. placebo	Not available	This ongoing study reported a benefit of clonazepam (80% of patients responded) over placebo (20% response) in adolescent panic disorder.
Selective serotonin reuptake inhibitors			
Black and Uhde (1994)	Fluoxetine vs. placebo	Yes	This small study in children with selective mutism, often complicated by social phobia, found a significant benefit of fluoxetine over placebo, although only for parent report.

(Gittelman-Klein and Klein 1971). Although the data from this study were quite striking in suggesting a role for imipramine in separation anxiety disorder, this positive view is tempered by the fact that the other studies, including another study by R. G. Klein et al. (1992) using an identical design, failed to replicate the findings. Moreover, when the failed replications are combined with recent concerns about the cardiotoxicity of TCAs in children, the weight of the evidence does not suggest TCAs to be a good first-line treatment for any of the disorders discussed in this chapter.

There are a few controlled trials of benzodiazepines in children with anxiety assessed before the major changes to the psychiatric nosology in DSM-III (see Allen et al. 1995 for review). Because these trials were usually conducted in children with other severe psychopathology beyond anxiety, the relevance of these data for the treatment of primary anxiety disorders remains unclear. Two other published controlled trials examined the efficacy of the high-potency benzodiazepines in childhood anxiety. These include one study of alprazolam (Simeon et al. 1992) and one study of clonazepam (Graae et al. 1994), both for overanxious disorder, with or without comorbidity. Bernstein et al. (1990) also included a group on alprazolam in their study of imipramine for separation anxiety disorder. None of these studies provided much evidence to support the use of these medications. One additional yet-to-be published study may provide data to support the use of high-potency benzodiazepines in adolescent panic disorder (see Kutcher et al. 1992).

Finally, one small controlled trial examined the efficacy of fluoxetine in selective mutism complicated by social phobia (Black and Uhde 1994). Although the results were generally encouraging, the study was small, and there was some inconsistency across informants as to the degree of improvement seen with the medication. Given suggestive data from three open trials in childhood anxiety disorders (Birmaher et al. 1994; Dummit et al. 1996; Fairbanks et al., in press), coupled with data from a recent study in childhood depression (Emslie et al. 1997), there is currently much interest in the potential utility of these medications in treating childhood anxiety.

In summary, there remain scant data from randomized, controlled trials to assist the clinician in the choice of a medication for treating children with anxiety disorders. Given this paucity of research, along with the data to suggest similarities in anxiety disorders of children and adults, the use of each class of medication in childhood anxiety disorders is discussed with extensive reference to the far more extensive database from studies with adults.

Using Medications to Treat Childhood Anxiety Disorders

Selective Serotonin Reuptake Inhibitors

Background.   The selective serotonin reuptake inhibitors (SSRIs) are unique medications in many respects. First, unlike older medicines whose utility was generally recognized through chance observations, these medications were developed specifically to target serotonin reuptake transporters localized on presynaptic serotonergic nerve terminals. Second, the side effect profile with SSRIs is generally more favorable than the other mainstays of anxiolytic therapy, benzodiazepines, and other antidepressant medications. Third, the widespread use of SSRIs has led to a new appreciation of the potential for drug-drug interactions when using pharmacological treatments for childhood psychiatric disorders.

The SSRIs are popular because of their record of efficacy in an array of conditions combined with a record of tolerability and safety. Currently, there are four SSRIs clinically available in the United States: fluoxetine, sertraline, paroxetine, and fluvoxamine. These medications are discussed as a group, and differences among the SSRIs are discussed when they impact on clinical care.

Indications.   Data from large randomized, controlled trials among adults demonstrate the efficacy of the SSRIs for the treatment of acute episodes of various anxiety disorders (Boyer 1995;

Greist et al. 1995; Marshall and Schneir 1996). For adults, beyond the data in obsessive-compulsive disorder, the most data are available for panic disorder (Boyer 1995; Coplan and Klein 1996), where the SSRIs are clinically considered to be equivalently effective treatments. The major differences among the SSRIs relate to differences in half-life and potential for drug-drug interactions, stemming from different effects of each SSRI on hepatic enzymes involved in medication metabolism. Fewer data exist on the efficacy of SSRIs for other adult anxiety disorders, though some emerging data suggest efficacy in social phobia (Marshall et al. 1996). As of this writing, no studies have been undertaken among adults with noncomorbid, "pure" generalized anxiety disorder. Despite relatively strong data on efficacy for most of the SSRIs, only paroxetine carries a Food and Drug Administration (FDA) indication for the treatment of panic disorder among adults.

For children, Black and Uhde (1994) provide the only data from a randomized, controlled trial of an SSRI for an anxiety disorder, reporting that fluoxetine appears helpful in selective mutism complicated by social phobia. As noted previously, data from three other open trials suggest efficacy in social phobia with or without selective mutism, overanxious or generalized anxiety disorder, and separation anxiety disorder (Birmaher et al. 1994; Dummit et al. 1996; Fairbanks et al. 1997).

Among both adults and children, the SSRIs are often chosen as a first-line treatment over medications such as the TCAs, monoamine oxidase inhibitors (MAOIs), and benzodiazepines. This preference derives from their excellent side effect profile, low abuse potential, and safety in overdose or in patients with concurrent medical illness.

Side effects. Although the lack of data from randomized, controlled trials in children clearly impacts conclusions on the efficacy of the SSRIs, this also limits conclusions on side effects. Without placebo-controlled data, side effects noted in open trials could be attributed to nonspecific effects of medication or to the somatic symptoms in anxiety disorders.

Data from controlled trials in childhood obsessive-compulsive disorder suggest that various mild side effects are relatively common with SSRIs, over and above rates seen with placebo (Riddle et al. 1992). These side effects usually include somatic complaints, such as headache, nausea, or gastrointestinal upset. SSRIs can also produce "activation" or even mild to moderate agitation in children and adolescents. Although there was some initial concern that this effect could occasionally be extreme, leading to frank mania, destructive behavior, or even suicidal ideation, the current view is that these medications are usually well tolerated, provided that the clinician starts with low doses and raises the dose relatively slowly. This view is supported by open trials in nearly 100 children and adolescents, where such extreme adverse reactions have not been seen.

In research among adults, the favorable side effect profile of the SSRIs is seen as one of the main advantages of these medications (see Preskorn 1996 for review). Most importantly for children, as well as adults, the SSRIs have few clinically relevant effects on the cardiovascular system, though more studies among children are needed. This feature stands in contrast to the TCAs, which can affect both cardiac conduction and blood pressure. One of the major complications of SSRI use among adults relates to the high rates of sexual side effects, well beyond rates in placebo, among both males and females. SSRIs can lead to changes in libido and can interfere with orgasm in both genders. There are few data on this issue in adolescents.

A number of other effects have been noted in adults but tend to occur less often and have been noted infrequently in children. These effects include urinary retention, increased sweating, visual disturbances, akathisia, dizziness, and fatigue. Effects on motor control have also been noted. Finally, SSRIs, like virtually all antidepressants, have been associated with the onset of mania in adults, as well as children and adolescents. It remains unclear whether the rate of SSRI-induced mania is lower than the rate of mania with other antidepressants.

Contraindications. The most frequent contraindications for SSRI therapy relate to the use of concurrent medications. The SSRIs inhibit various cytochrome P450 isozymes that are responsible for medication metabolism. This effect can produce toxic levels of concomitantly prescribed medications, in the face of appropriate doses, coadministered with SSRIs. Some specific examples of such interactions include the increase in TCA levels when coadministered with fluoxetine or sertraline, increases in theophylline or haloperidol levels when coadministered with fluvoxamine, and increases in phenytoin levels when coadministered with fluoxetine (Nemeroff et al. 1996; Preskorn 1996). For some medications, such as TCAs, SSRIs are only a relative contraindication, since the two medications can be concomitantly administered safely, provided that TCA levels are closely monitored. For other psychiatric medications, such as the MAOIs, combination therapy should be avoided, because serious adverse events, such as the serotonin syndrome, can result. In all cases, standard references of drug-drug interactions should be consulted before initiating SSRIs in a patient taking another medication concurrently (Ciraulo et al. 1995; Nemeroff et al. 1996; Preskorn 1996).

Toxicity.   Another key advantage to SSRIs is their safety, even in very large doses exceeding the usual therapeutic doses by 5- to 10-fold. Although overdoses in adults have been associated with agitation, vomiting, and rare seizures, as of this writing, no deaths have occurred from isolated SSRI overdose. The only two reported fluoxetine deaths followed overdose of at least 1,800 mg of fluoxetine in combination with other medications.

Clinical use.   SSRIs should be started at low doses in children and adolescents with anxiety disorders (approximately 5–10 mg of fluoxetine, 25 mg of fluvoxamine, 25 mg of sertraline, or 10 mg of paroxetine per day). The clinician should thoroughly review with children and parents the side effects of SSRIs, emphasizing the "activating" nature of the medications. The sexual side effects of the SSRIs should also be discussed with adolescent patients. The potential for inducing mania should be discussed with both children and their parents, noting the typical early signs of mania. Careful attention must be paid to any concurrently taken medications.

An initial SSRI dose is usually given in the morning to prevent insomnia. Since some patients experience drowsiness, they prefer to take an SSRI at night. The initial dose of an SSRI should be raised slowly, typically once or twice per week, and the dose should be carefully titrated to avoid extreme increases in anxiety related to each dose increase. After the first few weeks of treatment, the dose can be raised more quickly. In patients who continue to exhibit increased anxiety after a dose increase, the clinician should consider either a slower titration or even a dose reduction. Blood levels of SSRIs are not clinically useful, but it may be important to follow levels of medications that may be coadministered.

The anxiolytic effect of the SSRIs is usually not seen before 1 week, and the full effect might not be seen for many weeks, depending on how quickly the dose increases. Data from open studies and clinical experience suggest that effective doses in childhood anxiety disorders tend to be in the range for childhood and adult depression, with typical doses of approximately 20 mg/day for fluoxetine and paroxetine, 50–100 mg for sertraline, and 150 mg for fluvoxamine. Some younger children, however, may respond to even lower doses. Most of the SSRIs can be taken on a once-daily basis.

The choice of one or another SSRI should depend on two factors. First, in patients taking other medications, the choice of an SSRI should be based on the effect of the different SSRIs on the cytochrome P450 system, with care to avoid concomitant use of medications that might be affected adversely. Second, the clinician should consider the different half-lives of the SSRIs. For children and families in which compliance is an issue, the longer half-life of fluoxetine is a plus. Whereas patients might experience withdrawal or rebound anxiety after missing a dose of SSRIs with short half-lives, this effect rarely occurs with fluoxetine. For children who are complicated or treatment refractory, and for whom additional medications may be indicated, the SSRIs with shorter half-lives may be a better choice. Medications with shorter half-lives are also advantageous when there are concerns of inducing mania or increasing agitation in children. Because of the long half-life of fluoxetine, significant blood levels may persist for many weeks after drug discontinuation, which is problematic for patients who begin to show signs of mania or disinhibition.

Benzodiazepines

Background. The benzodiazepines have a chemical structure consisting of a benzene ring connected to a seven-member diazepine ring, with each specific benzodiazepine medication possessing unique substitutions at either of the two rings (Enna and Mohler 1987). Benzodiazepines are usually prescribed for either their anxiolytic effects, which occur at relatively low doses, or their soporific effects, which occur at relatively high doses. As anxiolytics, benzodiazepines can be categorized as high-potency (e.g., clonazepam and alprazolam) or low-potency (e.g., chlordiazepoxide, diazepam, and most others) medications. Potency of the benzodiazepines should not be confused with half-life of these medications—whereas potency refers to the effect of each medication on a target, half-life refers to the medication's metabolism time course. In general, high-potency benzodiazepines tend to have relatively short half-lives.

Indications. Among adults with generalized anxiety disorder, the efficacy of the benzodiazepines is well established (Schweizer 1995; Shader and Greenblatt 1995; Thompson 1996). There is also good evidence that benzodiazepines are effective in adult panic disorder, with the most complete data existing for the two high-potency benzodiazepines, clonazepam and alprazolam (Ballenger et al. 1988). The data remain equivocal from the three controlled studies using high-potency benzodiazepines in adult social phobia, with only one study finding clear superiority over placebo (Marshall and Schneier 1996). One controlled study examined the efficacy of alprazolam in adult PTSD, reporting some benefit for symptoms of anxiety in general but no specific benefit for PTSD-related symptoms (Marshall et al. 1996).

In contrast to these data among adults, there is considerably less information on the utility of benzodiazepines in childhood anxiety disorders. Moreover, as noted previously, in the data that do exist, there is far less evidence to support the use of these medications in children, as compared to adults, with anxiety disorders. None of the three recently published controlled trials provide strong data to support the use of these medications, particularly when the data on efficacy are weighed against the data on side effects.

Side effects.   The benzodiazepines are relatively devoid of cardiac and respiratory effects, causing respiratory depression only at moderate doses. The most troublesome, common side effects relate to central nervous system (CNS) depressive properties of these medications, which lead to complaints of fatigue, drowsiness, and difficulty concentrating in many patients. There is also evidence that the benzodiazepines impair memory and learning abilities, as well as motor coordination (Schweizer 1995). At least part of this deleterious effect derives from CNS depression. Given the cognitive demands of school and the adverse consequences of school failure, these side effects are particularly troublesome for children and adolescents.

Benzodiazepine use has been associated with exacerbation of major depressive disorder in children, adolescents, and adults, although the high-potency benzodiazepine alprazolam also has been noted to improve depressive symptoms among adults. Particularly in young children or among individuals with organic brain syndromes, benzodiazepines can precipitate disinhibition, which can be manifested as rage, agitation, and increased impulsivity. Finally, benzodiazepine use carries a significant risk of physical dependence and associated withdrawal symptoms, which relate to their abuse potential (Woods et al. 1992).

Contraindications.   Among individuals with a history of substance abuse, benzodiazepines should be used with extreme caution, if at all. Given the elevated rates of substance use experimentation during adolescence, this caveat is particularly important for child and adolescent psychiatrists. Underlying cognitive deficits or organic brain disease in a patient should also raise concerns in the clinician, given these medications' tendency to produce disinhibition or an exacerbation of cognitive deficits (Schweizer 1995). Care should be used in children with underlying lung diseases, such as asthma, because of the potential for respiratory depression associated with these medications. Finally, care should be taken with patients using other CNS depressants, given the potential for synergism with the benzodiazepines (Schweizer 1995; Woods et al. 1992).

Toxicity. Benzodiazepines are relatively safe in overdose. Overdose is of most concern when it occurs in the face of alcohol use or multiple drug ingestions.

Clinical use. As noted previously, few controlled data support the use of benzodiazepines in childhood anxiety disorders. In general, the medications should be considered only for children and adolescents without comorbid substance abuse or major depression who require immediate relief from paralyzing anxiety or for children and adolescents in which there are serious concerns about precipitation of mania.

Whereas the SSRIs usually require weeks to reduce anxiety, at least among adults, the anxiolytic and antipanic effects of the benzodiazepines are virtually immediate. Nevertheless, even in children or adolescents with no history of substance abuse, the risk of physical dependency to benzodiazepines must be carefully explained to both the patient and his or her parents. Moreover, because of this risk, benzodiazepines should be considered a second-line treatment for childhood anxiety disorders, and patients should be started on an SSRI whenever possible, using a benzodiazepine only in the early stages of treatment for immediate relief. Among children and adolescents with a history of mania or a strong history of mania in the family, it is worth considering the utility of a benzodiazepine. In contrast to virtually all other anxiolytics, the benzodiazepines tend not to induce mania. Some evidence shows a therapeutic benefit in patients with mania.

As with SSRIs, benzodiazepines should be started at a low dose. Usually clonazepam is the best first-line medication, since alprazolam is often associated with withdrawal anxiety. However, there is some anecdotal evidence that exacerbation of depression may be more frequent with clonazepam than with alprazolam. Many children do well on a very low dose of clonazepam, either 0.25 or 0.50 mg, taken one to two times per day, with an additional dose taken on an as-needed basis. Doses of up to 2 mg/day are typical in patients with severe anxiety. Care should be taken when titrating high-potency benzodiazepines such as clonazepam. In a study of childhood anxiety disorders, Graae et al. (1994) increased the dosage by 0.25 mg twice per week and found relatively high rates of irritability. For alprazolam, a 0.25- or 0.50-mg dose is also often used at the start of treatment, increased up to the 2- to 4-mg range, with some patients requiring more medication. Because of the shorter half-life of alprazolam, this medication may be needed more than twice a day, with an additional dose as needed.

The Azapirones

Background. The azapirones bind to the 5-HT_{1a} serotonin receptor, which is localized on both the cell body and terminals of serotonergic neurons and the dendrites of postsynaptic neurons receiving serotonergic innervation (Coplan and Klein 1996; Feighner 1987). These medications include three compounds currently available in either the United States or Europe—buspirone, gepirone, and ipsapirone—as well as a number of experimental compounds. Enthusiasm for these medications followed from the increased appreciation of the role of serotonin in anxiety, effects of these medications on animal models of anxiety, and the favorable side effect profile for these medications. This initial enthusiasm, however, has not generally translated into acceptance of the azapirones as a mainstay of treatment for anxiety disorder beyond generalized anxiety disorder. Studies among adults document efficacy in generalized anxiety but not other anxiety disorders. There are no known published randomized, controlled trials in children and no known studies that are nearing completion.

Indications.   Among adults, buspirone has been established as an effective treatment for generalized anxiety disorder and has received FDA approval for this indication (Feighner 1987; Shader and Greenblatt 1995). Like the response of most adult anxiety disorders to SSRIs, the response of generalized anxiety disorder to buspirone is manifested only after a number of days. In contrast to the SSRIs, a number of studies clearly point to the poor efficacy of azapirones in adult panic disorder (Coplan and Klein 1996). Similarly, open data suggest that azapirones might be beneficial in social phobia, but the only controlled trial, which was for specific social phobia, suggested a lack of efficacy (Marshall and Schneier 1996).

Side effects.   Though there are no controlled data on side effects in children or adolescents, studies among adults show the azapirones to be relatively free of side effects. In particular, they lack the abuse liability, tolerance, risk for withdrawal syndromes, and psychomotor or cognitive effects of the benzodiazepines; they also lack the marked effects on the cardiovascular system associated with TCAs. Azapirones have been associated with gastrointestinal upset, headaches, and occasional complaints of restlessness, nervousness, and sleep disturbance. These symptoms are rarely severe enough to interfere with the use of the medications. Compared to the benzodiazepines, the azapirones tend to be associated with less drowsiness, cognitive side effects, and fatigue but more nervousness and gastrointestinal complaints.

Contraindications and toxicity.   The major contraindication to azapirones relates to concomitant medication use. For example, the azapirones should be used cautiously with MAOIs because there are reports of blood pressure elevation associated with this combination.

Clinical use.   Because there are limited data from open studies, and no available data from randomized, controlled trials on the utility of azapirones in childhood anxiety, data to support the utility of these medications in childhood anxiety disorders derive from studies among adults. In adults, the main disadvantages to the azapirones is their delayed onset of anxiolysis and narrow range of symptoms they target. With regard to dosing in adults for buspirone, the only azapirone available in the United States, an initial 5-mg dose, taken twice a day, is typically used, with 5-mg increases two to three times per week. The usual effective dose is in the 30- to 40-mg range for adults. It should be noted that the azapirones also have some efficacy in adult major depression but are not good treatments for panic attacks. Given the lack of data among children and adolescents, these medications are not considered first-line medications for the treatment of childhood anxiety.

Tricyclic Antidepressants

Background.   The efficacy of TCAs in adult anxiety and depression was discovered by chance observation. Efficacy for depression was noted during trials for psychosis, while efficacy for anxiety disorders was noted in the context of treating anxious patients with a variety of medications.

The TCAs share a common chemical structure, consisting of two benzene rings joined by a seven-member ring with either a nitrogen or carbon atom. These medications are subclassified according to the structure of the terminal amine group as either tertiary amine TCAs (imipramine, amitriptyline, clomipramine, and doxepin) or secondary amine TCAs (desipramine, nortriptyline, protriptyline, and amoxapine). Two of the secondary amine TCAs (desipramine and nortriptyline) are demethylated tertiary amine TCAs (imipramine and amitriptyline). Although the TCAs were once considered the first-line treatment for a number of adult anxiety disorders, they have been used less frequently in recent years among adults and even less frequently among children and adolescents. This reduction in use derives predominantly from the more favorable side effect profile of newer medications, coupled with equivocal data on efficacy, at least among children and adolescents.

Indications. Beyond the data on the use of clomipramine in childhood obsessive-compulsive disorder (DeVeaugh-Geiss et al. 1992), the data reviewed earlier on the use of TCAs in childhood anxiety disorders are equivocal, at best. These data stand in contrast to the data among adults, where the medications have a solid foundation supporting their efficacy. Panic disorder, which is very rare in children, represents the most frequently noted adult anxiety disorder for which TCAs are prescribed (Mavissakalian and Perel 1995; Pollack and Smoller 1995; Shader and Greenblatt 1995). Two randomized, controlled trials demonstrate the efficacy of TCAs in adult generalized anxiety disorder (Rickels et al. 1993). Although there have been relatively few controlled trials of pharmacotherapy for adult PTSD, at least four studies examined the efficacy of TCAs, with somewhat mixed results (Marshall et al. 1996). Finally, TCAs are not considered a first-line treatment for adult social phobia, of either the specific or generalized nature (Liebowitz et al. 1992; Marshall and Schneier 1996), where there are far better data on efficacy for the MAOIs, as well as for the SSRIs.

Side effects. The main limitation to the use of TCAs relates to their side effect profile, particularly because of their impact on cardiac conduction. These effects, when coupled with the equivocal data on efficacy for childhood disorders, make the TCAs a secondary treatment for childhood anxiety disorders besides obsessive-compulsive disorder.

The TCAs also possess other less dangerous but troublesome side effects, including anticholinergic effects, which are particularly common with the tertiary amines, producing symptoms such as drowsiness, lethargy, urinary retention, dry mouth, constipation, blurred vision, and gastrointestinal upset. The effects of the TCAs on histamine can further exacerbate cognitive complaints.

Contraindications. The potential for cardiac toxicity warrants a generally cautious approach to TCA use in children. Beyond this general issue in all children or adolescents, other serious contraindications to TCA use involve either underlying cardiac disease or a serious concern with potential overdose. TCAs should be avoided in these scenarios. Clinicians should be wary of drug-drug interactions when using TCAs, which can take many forms. Concomitant use with medications such as the SSRIs, which inhibit cytochrome P450 activity, can produce toxic levels of TCAs, even when prescribed in low doses. Concomitant use of other anticholinergics can precipitate an anticholinergic delirium or other serious anticholinergic effects, such as urinary retention. Finally, concomitant use with other sedative medications (e.g., benzodiazepines and antihistamines) or with medications that affect the cardiac system (e.g., neuroleptics and beta-blockers) can lead to CNS or cardiac toxicity, despite the use of low medication doses.

Toxicity.   As noted previously, the most serious toxicity associated with the TCAs derives from these medications' effect on cardiac conduction. Overdoses with TCAs can produce life-threatening arrhythmias. That the difference between a therapeutic versus a toxic dose of the medication is small (i.e., a narrow therapeutic window) is of particular concern. An overdose of 1 g of TCAs, which is usually less than 1 week's worth of medication, is considered potentially lethal.

Clinical use.   TCAs should be considered only in patients with extreme anxiety, where other medications have either failed or are not a therapeutic option. Before starting a TCA in a child with an anxiety disorder, a normal electrocardiogram must be obtained, and a repeat cardiogram should be obtained after each dosage change. It is particularly important to monitor conduction parameters, including the P-R, QRS, and QT_c intervals, during treatment. As with the SSRIs, TCAs should be started in low dosages and raised relatively slowly. In the most recent trial of imipramine for separation anxiety disorder, R. G. Klein et al. (1992) started with a 25-mg/day dose, increased to 50 mg/day at day 4, and then titrated to a dose of 5 mg/kg. Although there are insufficient data on the utility of drug levels in treating childhood anxiety disorders, studies among adults suggest that the combined level of imipramine and desipramine should be at least in the 110- to 140-ng/ml range for effective treatment of panic disorder (Mavissakalian and Perel 1995). In children, blood levels should be followed closely to prevent accumulation of these compounds.

Other Medications

A variety of other medications are occasionally used in the treatment of childhood anxiety disorders. Although there are limited data to support the utility of the preceding medications, there are virtually no data for the following medications.

Beta-blockers. Beta-blockers are not an approved treatment for any psychiatric disorder, though they have been used to treat various conditions, including anxiety disorders. Studies among adults show these medications to exhibit little efficacy in either panic disorder or generalized anxiety disorder. There has been interest in their use for PTSD, but no definitive data suggest efficacy among either children or adults. Perhaps the only established role for beta-blockers with anxiety disorders is in performance anxiety, where the only available data are in adults.

Alpha-2 agonists. There has been a theoretical interest in alpha-2 agonists, which include clonidine, for the treatment of various anxiety disorders. One model of panic-related anxiety focuses on the role of locus coeruleus hyperactivity. Alpha-2 agonists increase the inhibitory tone on the locus coeruleus, which could be of potential benefit. Following from this theoretical view, the clinical utility of these medications was most firmly supported by findings in narcotic withdrawal. Controlled trials in adult anxiety disorders suggest modest benefits of clonidine, but the side effect profile limits the usefulness of this medication, and there are no data among children and adolescents, where the medications have been used to treat tics and disruptive behavior disorders.

Non-SSRI/tricyclic serotonergic/noradrenergic compounds.
Trazodone is a serotonin agonist that induces anxiety in challenge tests with adults with panic disorder as well as patients with obsessive-compulsive disorder. Although no controlled data exist on the use of this agent in childhood anxiety, there is evidence of efficacy for adult generalized anxiety disorder (Rickels et al. 1993). Trazodone is without marked effects on cardiac conduction but can cause orthostatic hypotension. Priapism is a rare but notable side effect of trazodone, and the risk for priapism must be discussed with males. A number of other compounds that share properties with older medications that effectively treat anxiety disorders have been developed or are in the late stages of clinical testing (Shader and Greenblatt 1995). For example, venlafaxine, a mixed serotonin/noradrenaline reuptake inhibitor, may eventually prove beneficial in treating anxiety disorders, as may nefazoone, a similar compound that also possesses 5-HT_2 antagonism. Preliminary data for a third new compound, ritanserin, which has strong 5-HT_2 antagonism, do not suggest marked efficacy in adult anxiety disorders. Other serotonergic medications with possible effects on anxiety include the 5-HT_3 antagonist ondansetron. Preliminary data among adults suggest efficacy in generalized anxiety disorder.

Conclusion

We have reviewed the clinical features and psychopharmacology of childhood anxiety disorders. Given the limited available psychopharmacological data on childhood anxiety disorders besides obsessive-compulsive disorder, this chapter integrates a review of research on the similarities between childhood and adult anxiety disorders with a summary of the pharmacological literature in adult anxiety disorders. The wealth of data among adults can be used to justify a rational pharmacological approach to childhood disorders. Nevertheless, this pharmacological approach must be considered tentative, given the paucity of controlled data in children. Research on the validity and psychopharmacology of childhood depression emphasizes the importance of conducting independent clinical trials directly in children and adolescents with various types of anxiety disorders. Given the prevalence of childhood anxiety disorders and their associated long-term risks, such trials are of critical importance.

References

Allen AJ, Leonard HL, Swedo SE: Current knowledge of medications for the treatment of childhood anxiety disorders. J Am Acad Child Adolesc Psychiatry 34:976–986, 1995

American Psychiatric Association: Diagnostic and Statistical Manual of Mental Disorders, 3rd Edition. Washington, DC, American Psychiatric Association, 1980

American Psychiatric Association: Diagnostic and Statistical Manual of Mental Disorders, 3rd Edition, Revised. Washington, DC, American Psychiatric Association, 1987

American Psychiatric Association: Diagnostic and Statistical Manual of Mental Disorders, 4th Edition. Washington, DC, American Psychiatric Association, 1994

Ballenger J, Burrows G, DuPont R, et al: Alprazolam in panic disorder and agoraphobia: results from a multicenter trial, I: efficacy in short-term treatment. Arch Gen Psychiatry 45:413–422, 1988

Barlow DH: Anxiety and Its Disorders: The Nature and Treatment of Anxiety and Panic. New York, Guilford, 1988

Beidel DC, Turner SM: At risk for anxiety, I: psychopathology in the offspring of anxious parents. J Am Acad Child Adolesc Psychiatry 36:918–924, 1997

Berney T, Kolvin I, Bhate SR, et al: School phobia: a therapeutic trial with clomipramine and short-term outcome. Br J Psychiatry 138:110–118, 1981

Bernstein GA, Garfinkel BD, Borchardt CM: Comparative studies of pharmacotherapy for school refusal. J Am Acad Child Adolesc Psychiatry 29:773–781, 1990

Birmaher B, Waterman GS, Ryan N, et al: Fluoxetine for childhood anxiety disorders. J Am Acad Child Adolesc Psychiatry 33:993–999, 1994

Black B, Uhde TW: Treatment of elective mutism with fluoxetine: a double-blind placebo controlled study. J Am Acad Child Adolesc Psychiatry 33:1000–1006, 1994

Boyer W: Serotonin uptake inhibitors are superior to imipramine and alprazolam in alleviating panic attacks: a meta-analysis. Int Clin Psychopharmacol 10:45–49, 1995

Breslau N, Davis GC, Prabucki K: Searching for evidence on the validity of generalized anxiety disorder: psychopathology in children of anxious mothers. Psychiatry Res 20:285–297, 1987

Ciraulo DA, Shader RI, Greenblatt DJ, et al: Drug Interactions in Psychiatry, 2nd Edition. Baltimore, MD, Williams & Wilkins, 1995

Coplan JD, Klein DF: Pharmacological probes in panic disorder, in Advances in the Neurobiology of Anxiety Disorders. Edited by Westenberg HGM, Den Boer JA, Murphy DL. New York, Wiley, 1996, pp 173–196

Costello EJ, Angold A: Epidemiology, in Anxiety Disorders in Children and Adolescents. Edited by March JS. New York, Guilford, 1995, pp 109–124

DeVeaugh-Geiss J, Moroz G, Biederman J, et al: Clomipramine hydrochloride in childhood and adolescent obsessive-compulsive disorder: a multicenter trial. J Am Acad Child Adolesc Psychiatry 31:45–49, 1992

Dummit ES, Klein RG, Tancer NK, et al: Fluoxetine treatment of children with selective mutism: an open trial. J Am Acad Child Adolesc Psychiatry 35:615–621, 1996

Eaton WW, Dryman A, Weissman MM: Panic and phobia, in Psychiatric Disorders in America: The Epidemiologic Catchment Area Study. Edited by Robins LN, Regier DA. New York, Free Press, 1991, pp 180–203

Emslie GJ, Weinberg WA, Kowatch RA, et al: Fluoxetine treatment of depressed children and adolescents. Arch Gen Psychiatry 54:1031–1037, 1997

Enna SJ, Mohler H: Gamma amino butyric acid receptors and their association with benzodiazepine recognition sites, in Psychopharmacology: The Third Generation of Progress. Edited by Meltzer HY. New York, Raven, 1987, pp 265–272

Fairbanks JM, Pine DS, Tancer NK, et al: Open fluoxetine treatment of childhood anxiety disorders. Journal of Child and Adolescent Psychopharmacology 7:17–29, 1997

Feighner JP: Buspirone in the long-term treatment of generalized anxiety disorder. J Clin Psychiatry 48(suppl):3–6, 1987

Fyer AJ, Mannuzza S, Chapman TF, et al: Specificity in familial aggregation of phobic disorders. Arch Gen Psychiatry 52:564–573, 1995

Gittelman-Klein R, Klein DF: Controlled imipramine treatment of school phobia. Arch Gen Psychiatry 25:204–207, 1971

Goldstein RB, Wickramaratne PJ, Horwath E, et al: Familial aggregation and phenomenology of "early"-onset (at or before age 20 years) panic disorder. Arch Gen Psychiatry 54:271–278, 1997

Graae F, Milner J, Rizzotto L, et al: Clonazepam in childhood anxiety disorders. Journal of the American Academy of Child Psychiatry 33:372–376, 1994

Greist JH, Jefferson JW, Kobak KA, et al: Efficacy and tolerability of serotonin transport inhibitors in obsessive compulsive disorder: a meta-analysis. Arch Gen Psychiatry 52:53–60, 1995

Gurley D, Cohen P, Pine DS, et al: The comorbidity of anxiety disorders and depression in a large community sample of youth. J Affective Disord 39:191–200, 1996

Ianlongo N, Edelshon G, Werthamer-Larsson L, et al: The significance of self-reported anxious symptoms in first grade children: prediction to anxious symptoms and adaptive functioning in fifth grade. J Child Psychol Psychiatry 36:427–437, 1995

Kendall PC: Treating anxiety disorders in children: results of a randomized clinical trial. J Consult Clin Psychol 62:100–110, 1994

Kendler KS, Walters EE, Neale MC, et al: The structure of the genetic and environmental risk factors for six major psychiatric disorders in women. Arch Gen Psychiatry 52:374–383, 1995

Klein DF: False suffocation alarms, spontaneous panics, and related conditions: an integrative hypothesis. Arch Gen Psychiatry 50:307–317, 1993

Klein RG: Anxiety disorders, in Child and Adolescent Psychiatry: Modern Approaches, 3rd Edition. Edited by Rutter M, Taylor E, Hersov L. London, Blackwell Scientific, 1995a, pp 351–374

Klein RG: Is panic disorder associated with childhood separation anxiety disorder? Clin Neuropharmacology 18(suppl):S7–S14, 1995b

Klein RG, Koplewicz HS, Kanner A: Imipramine treatment of children with separation anxiety disorder. J Am Acad Child Adolesc Psychiatry 31:21–28, 1992

Kutcher SP, Reiter S, Gardner DM, et al: Pharmacotherapy of anxiety disorders in children and adolescents. Psychiatr Clin North Am 15:41–68, 1992

Last CG, Hersen M, Kazdin AE, et al: Anxiety disorders in children and their families. Arch Gen Psychiatry 48:928–934, 1991

Last CG, Perrin S, Hersen M, et al: A prospective study of childhood anxiety disorders. J Am Acad Child Adolesc Psychiatry 35:1502–1510, 1996

Liebowitz MR, Schneir F, Campeas R, et al: Phenelzine vs. atenolol in social phobia: a placebo controlled comparison. Arch Gen Psychiatry 49:290–300, 1992

Magee WJ, Eaton WW, Wittchen H, et al: Agoraphobia, simple phobia, and social phobia in the National Comorbidity Survey. Arch Gen Psychiatry 53:159–168, 1996

Marks IM: Fears, Phobias, and Rituals: Panic, Anxiety, and Their Disorders. New York, Oxford University Press, 1988

Marshall RD, Schneier FR: An algorithm for the pharmacotherapy of social phobia. Psychiatric Annals 26:210–216, 1996

Marshall RD, Stein DJ, Liebowitz MR, et al: A pharmacotherapy algorithm in the treatment of posttraumatic stress disorder. Psychiatric Annals 26:217–226, 1996

Mavissakalian MR, Perel JM: Imipramine treatment of panic disorder with agoraphobia: dose ranging and plasma level-response relationships. Am J Psychiatry 152:673–682, 1995

Mrazek DA: Psychiatric complications of pediatric asthma. Annals of Allergy 69:285–290, 1992

Nemeroff CB, DeVane CL, Pollock BG: Newer antidepressants and the cytochrome P450 system. Am J Psychiatry 153:311–320, 1996

Pike A, Reiss D, Hetherington EM, et al: Using MZ differences in the search for nonshared environmental effects. J Child Psychol Psychiatry 37:695–704, 1996

Pine DS, Cohen P, Brook J: Emotional problems during youth as predictors of stature during early adulthood: results from a prospective epidemiologic study. Pediatrics 97:856–863, 1996

Pine DS, Cohen P, Gurley D, et al: The relationship between anxiety and depression in adolescence and early-adulthood. Arch Gen Psychiatry 55:56–66, 1998

Pine DS, Coplan JD, Papp LA, et al: Ventilatory physiology in children and adolescents with anxiety disorders. Arch Gen Psychiatry (in press)

Pine DS, Weese-Mayer DE, Silvestri JM, et al: Anxiety and congenital central hypoventilation syndrome. Am J Psychiatry 151:864–870, 1994

Pollack MH, Smoller JW: The longitudinal course and outcome of panic disorder. Psychiatr Clin North Am 18:785–801, 1995

Preskorn SH: Clinical Pharmacology of Selective Serotonin Re-Uptake Inhibitors. Caddo, OK, Professional Communications, 1996

Rickels K, Downing R, Schweizer E, et al: Antidepressant and the treatment of generalized anxiety disorder: a placebo-controlled comparison of imipramine, trazodone, and diazepam. Arch Gen Psychiatry 50:884–895, 1993

Riddle MA, Scahill L, King RA, et al: Double-blind, crossover trial of fluoxetine and placebo in children and adolescents with obsessive-compulsive disorder. J Am Acad Child Adolesc Psychiatry 31:1062–1069, 1992

Schweizer E: Generalized anxiety disorder: longitudinal course and pharmacologic treatment. Psychiatr Clin North Am 18:843–856, 1995

Shader RI, Greenblatt DJ: The pharmacotherapy of acute anxiety: a mini-update, in Psychopharmacology: The Fourth Generation of Progress. Edited by Bloom FE, Kupfer DJ. New York, Raven, 1995, pp 1341–1348

Silove D, Manicavasagar V, O'Connell D, et al: Genetic factors in early separation anxiety: implications for the genesis of adult anxiety disorders. Acta Psychiatr Scand 92:17–74, 1995

Simeon JG, Ferguson HB, Knott V, et al: Clinical, cognitive, and neurophysiological effects of alprazolam in children and adolescents with overanxious and avoidant disorders. J Am Acad Child Adolesc Psychiatry 31:29–33, 1992

Thapar A, McGuffin P: A twin study of antisocial and neurotic symptoms in childhood. Psychol Med 26:1111–1118, 1996

Thompson PM: Generalized anxiety disorder treatment algorithm. Psychiatric Annals 26:227–232, 1996

Wambalt MZ, Weintraub P, Krafchick D, et al: Psychiatric family history in adolescents with severe asthma. J Am Acad Child Adolesc Psychiatry 35:1042–1049, 1996

Warner V, Mufson L, Weissman MM: Offspring at low and high risk for depression and anxiety: mechanisms of psychiatric disorder. J Am Acad Child Adolesc Psychiatry 34:786–797, 1995

Woods JH, Katz JL, Winger G: Benzodiazepines: use, abuse, and consequences. Pharmacol Rev 44:155–186, 1992

Chapter 6

Eating Disorders

Laurel E. S. Mayer, M.D., and B. Timothy Walsh, M.D.

In the last several decades, compelling evidence has emerged documenting the utility of pharmacological interventions for a variety of psychiatric disorders. The symptoms of many of these illnesses, particularly mood disturbances and obsessive-compulsive disorder, overlap symptomatically with the eating disorders. However, the role of medication in eating disorders remains, in general, less clearly established. Clinical trials of medication have been particularly disheartening for the treatment of anorexia nervosa. The efficacy of antidepressant agents in studies of the treatment of bulimia nervosa has been more encouraging; however, because forms of short-term, focused psychotherapy are at least equally effective and may have superior long-term benefits, the precise role of medication in the treatment of bulimia nervosa remains unclear. Additionally, despite the fact that anorexia nervosa and bulimia nervosa typically have their onset during adolescence and early adulthood, the overwhelming majority of medication trials have been conducted among patients 18 years of age or older. Thus, the results of these trials may not be generalizable to the pediatric population. In this chapter we review clinical studies of medications for the treatment of the eating disorders anorexia nervosa and bulimia nervosa, with emphasis on controlled trials and, when available, studies of adolescent populations.

Anorexia Nervosa

Anorexia nervosa is a psychiatric illness that predominantly affects adolescent and young women. It is associated with distortions of thinking and perceptions about shape and body image, leaving the teenager or young adult thinking she is fat and disgusting. In the most severe cases, the relentless cycle of dieting and weight loss can result in death.

The currently recommended treatments for anorexia nervosa employ an atheoretical, eclectic, multidisciplinary approach. Individual and family psychotherapies with cognitive-behavioral components are the primary modalities of treatment, with pharmacotherapy often used as an adjunct (American Psychiatric Association 1993; Garner and Garfinkel 1997). Although recent advances have provided us with increasing knowledge about various neurotransmitter and neuroendocrine disturbances, the etiology of anorexia nervosa remains elusive. Therefore, despite these recent advances, behavioral and psychosocial treatments remain the standard, and there are only hints that pharmacological interventions may have some use in the therapy of anorexia nervosa.

Methodological Issues in Studies of Anorexia Nervosa

The efficacy of medications in anorexia nervosa has been studied in a limited number of controlled trials. These trials have been conducted predominantly in low-weight, hospitalized patients, and the primary goal has been to enhance the rate of weight gain. One of the methodological limitations of these studies is that, as inpatients, the subjects are typically concurrently engaged in a behavioral treatment program focused on weight gain, and thus additional benefit of medication may be difficult to detect. Furthermore, there is substantial clinical and biologic heterogeneity among patients with anorexia nervosa. It is possible that only patients with specific, as yet unidentified characteristics respond to pharmacological intervention. Thus, trials conducted including patients with a variety of characteristics may obscure the benefits of the medication. It may be helpful, in future studies, to focus on subgroups, such as patients with the restricting or binge-purge subtypes, patients with short duration of illness, or patients who have already attained a certain level of weight restoration.

Antipsychotic Medication

The earliest systematic studies on the use of medication in the treatment of anorexia nervosa were performed by Dally and Sargant (1960, 1966). They administered chlorpromazine in doses of up to 1,600 mg/day, often in combination with insulin, to 30 hospitalized patients with anorexia nervosa. They compared the rate of weight gain in this group to that of 27 patients who had been treated previously on the same unit without medication. Those treated with chlorpromazine gained weight faster and were discharged sooner than those who had not received medication, but the chlorpromazine-treated patients also experienced significantly more side effects. Purging developed in 45%, compared to only 12% of nonmedicated patients. Of even more concern, 5 of 30 patients (17%) experienced grand mal seizures. On long-term follow-up, there was no significant difference in the two groups' weights or general outcome.

The only other studies of the efficacy of antipsychotic medication were conducted almost two decades later. Based on a theory proposed by Barry and Klawans (1976) that the physical activity often seen in anorexia nervosa might reflect increased dopamine transmission, Vandereycken and Pierloot (1982) carried out a randomized, double-blind, placebo-controlled study of the dopamine antagonist pimozide. Of 17 hospitalized patients, 8 received pimozide (4 or 6 mg/day) for 3 weeks and then were crossed over to receive placebo for 3 weeks; the remaining 9 patients received placebo first, followed by pimozide. Both groups were simultaneously engaged in a behaviorally oriented weight gain program. Although there was a trend for patients to have higher mean daily weight gain on pimozide than on placebo ($P = .07$), patients' attitudes as rated by staff were minimally altered.

The same group subsequently conducted a double-blind, placebo-controlled crossover study of the antipsychotic sulpiride. Eighteen hospitalized women with anorexia nervosa received 3 weeks each of sulpiride and placebo while daily weight gain and psychological measures were collected. Overall, no statistically significant differences were seen in either weight gain or patients' eating attitudes and behaviors (Vandereycken 1984).

Therefore, the controlled studies of the use of antipsychotic medications are few in number and provide little evidence that these agents substantially assist treatment. Given their potential for both short- and long-term side effects, antipsychotic medications are not recommended for the standard treatment of anorexia nervosa. However, their use may be considered for treatment-refractory patients who have not responded to conventional approaches.

Antidepressant Medication

Two major observations prompted clinical trials of antidepressant medications for the treatment of anorexia nervosa. First, patients with anorexia nervosa often manifest symptoms of depression, if not the full syndrome of major depression, including depressed mood, low energy, poor concentration, loss of interest, and a preference for social isolation. In addition, it was thought that the often unwanted side effect of weight gain from tricyclic antidepressants (TCAs) might be of benefit in underweight patients with anorexia nervosa. The controlled trials of antidepressant medications, however, are generally disappointing.

Lacey and Crisp (1980) examined the effect of clomipramine (50 mg/day) on the rate of weight gain. The eight patients on active medication reported significantly increased appetite while taking this very low dose, but their weight gain was slower than that of the placebo-treated patients. No differences were seen between the groups on long-term (1 and 4 years) follow-up.

The TCA amitriptyline was studied by Biederman et al. (1985). Twenty-five subjects, most of whom were inpatients, were divided into two groups: 11 were randomly assigned to receive amitriptyline, and 14 were randomly assigned to receive placebo. Eighteen patients who were otherwise eligible refused to take medication and served as an additional comparison group. Amitriptyline was administered up to a maximum dose of 175 mg/day. While blood levels of amitriptyline were followed and varied widely, there was no correlation between blood level and improvement in symptoms. Overall, the amitriptyline group reported increased side effects, and there was no suggestion of a significant difference among the three groups with respect to mood, weight gain, or body perception.

A second trial of amitriptyline (Halmi et al. 1986) compared its utility to that of cyproheptadine (a serotonin antagonist) and of placebo among 72 hospitalized patients. At a maximum daily dose of amitriptyline of 160 mg, side effects were minor. Although the mean number of days needed to reach target weight was lower for both medication groups (32 ± 17 days for amitriptyline, 36 ± 20 days for cyproheptadine, and 45 ± 18 days for placebo), other outcome measures showed no benefit of amitriptyline over placebo. A decrease in depressive symptoms was reported, but this improvement appeared to be more closely related to weight gain than to medication.

These studies of amitriptyline in anorexia nervosa were conducted well before the recent concern surrounding the possible association between TCAs and sudden death in children and adolescents (Wilens et al. 1996, see also Chapter 3 in this text). Despite the fact that anorexia nervosa is associated with a variety of cardiac disturbances, including prolongation of the Q-T interval, no serious cardiac complications were associated with the use of amitriptyline in the studies of either Biederman et al. (1985) or Halmi et al. (1986). Nonetheless, the recent concern about the safety of TCAs in young people and the lack of evidence supporting utility suggest that TCAs should be rarely used, at most, in underweight patients with anorexia nervosa.

The selective serotonin reuptake inhibitors (SSRIs) have largely replaced previously available antidepressants in general psychiatric practice, in large part because of the superior side effect profile of the newer agents. However, the efficacy of SSRIs in the treatment of anorexia nervosa is only now being studied. Ferguson (1987) published a case report of successful treatment of a woman with fluoxetine who had previously been difficult to treat because of the development of side effects on other medications. Gwirtsman (1990) reported results of an open trial of fluoxetine in six patients with anorexia nervosa. All showed improvement in depressive symptoms and an increase in weight. Our own group at Columbia has recently completed what we believe to be the only placebo-controlled trial of fluoxetine among underweight patients with anorexia nervosa. Preliminary analysis of these data suggests that the impact of fluoxetine, provided in the context of a behaviorally oriented inpatient program, was disappointing (Attia et al., in press).

The studies of antidepressant medication described previously all focused on what might be termed the *acute* treatment of patients with anorexia nervosa. All of the patients in these studies were underweight and were receiving psychosocial interventions to promote weight gain, and most were hospitalized. Recently, investigators have begun to focus on a different problem in the treatment of anorexia nervosa, namely, the high rate of relapse after weight restoration. The most provocative data come from a preliminary report of Kaye and colleagues (1997). In this study, 35 patients, all of whom were classed as having the restricting subtype of anorexia nervosa and who had regained to near-normal weight during an inpatient stay, were randomized to either fluoxetine or placebo and discharged to the community for continuing psychosocial care. The patients who received fluoxetine had a significantly lower rate of relapse than those receiving placebo. On the other hand, a naturalistic follow-up study by Strober et al. (in press) suggested little benefit from fluoxetine. As part of an ongoing, longitudinal study, 66 patients were followed after weight restoration and discharge from an inpatient unit. Thirty-three patients received up to a maximum target dose of 60 mg of fluoxetine, begun during their inpatient stay, and were compared to 33 case-control patients receiving no medication. Although follow-up treatment was not standardized, all patients were engaged in at least weekly psychotherapy, with the addition of family therapy and dietary counseling as recommended. Assessments were made during face-to-face interviews performed by the research staff at 6-month intervals for 2 years. No patient was lost to follow-up, and compliance with medication was very high, with only four patients discontinuing medication by the end of the second-year follow-up visit. Overall, the authors found no significant difference between the fluoxetine-treated and control groups on measures of compensatory behaviors, need for rehospitalization, and tendency to drop below target weight. Although interpretation of these data is limited because of the naturalistic design of this study, they cannot be summarily dismissed. Thus, whether treatment with fluoxetine is helpful in preventing relapse remains an active and important question for further research.

Cyproheptadine

Central nervous system (CNS) serotonergic activity is well known to be involved in the control of eating behavior. Injection of serotonergic agonists into the hypothalamus generally produces a reduction of food intake, and, conversely, the injection of serotonin antagonists results in increased food intake. Cyproheptadine is an antihistamine used in the treatment of allergic conditions that also possesses central serotonin antagonist properties. When used to treat pruritus associated with allergic reactions, cyproheptadine has been associated with weight gain in non-eating-disordered patients. In an attempt to capitalize on this side effect, investigators have examined the utility of cyproheptadine in anorexia nervosa.

There have been three controlled trials to date. In an 8-week trial (Vigersky and Loriaux 1977), 13 outpatients who received 12 mg/day of cyproheptadine were compared to 11 patients who received placebo. There was no significant difference between the groups. Goldberg et al. (1979) performed a double-blind, placebo-controlled, randomized trial of cyproheptadine in doses up to 32 mg/day among hospitalized patients. Although again there was no significant difference in weight gain between the active medication and control groups, cyproheptadine appeared to induce significant weight gain in a subpopulation of patients who had a "more severe form" of the illness.

The third study of cyproheptadine was that by Halmi et al.

(1986), referred to earlier. Although time to reach target weight was significantly shorter in the group treated with cyproheptadine (32 mg/day) compared to placebo, overall there was no significant difference in weight gain between the active medication and placebo groups. The authors did note, however, a provocative relationship between binge-purge subtype and response to medication. For restricting patients, cyproheptadine enhanced the rate of weight gain, whereas for patients with binge eating and/or purging, cyproheptadine slowed weight gain. These results are consistent with the notion that restricting behavior is associated with a relatively hyperserotonergic state, which is counteracted by a serotonin antagonist, while binge eating behavior is associated with a hyposerotonergic state, which is worsened by a serotonin antagonist.

Thus, despite a reasonable theoretical basis for postulating a possible role for cyproheptadine, the available data do not suggest that this agent has a major impact on the symptoms of anorexia nervosa, and it is used infrequently by specialized eating disorder programs at present.

Lithium

Because of its commonly noted side effect of weight gain and its efficacy as a mood stabilizer, lithium as a treatment for anorexia nervosa was assessed in a single placebo-controlled trial (Gross et al. 1981). The authors noted that the average weight gain of the lithium-treated group appeared greater than that of the placebo group during the latter half of the 4-week trial. Interpretation of these findings, however, is severely limited because of the very small sample size ($N = 16$) and brief duration (4 weeks) of the trial.

Tetrahydrocannabinol

Tetrahydrocannabinol (THC) is the active ingredient found in cannabis leaves and can be purified and administered in pill form. Given the potent appetite-stimulating and antiemetic properties of THC, Gross et al. (1983) conducted a study testing its benefit in daily oral use. Results of a 4-week, double-blind, crossover study in 11 patients comparing oral THC to diazepam showed no significant effect on food intake or weight. Significant differences were found on measures of somatization, interpersonal sensitivity, and sleep disturbance, with the THC group reporting more symptoms than the diazepam group. Three patients receiving THC experienced severe dysphoric mood, paranoia, and a feeling of being out of control and dropped out of the study prematurely.

Cisapride

Given the frequent somatic complaints of gastric fullness and bloating in patients with anorexia nervosa, investigators wondered about the efficacy of prokinetic agents in relieving these symptoms and allowing increased food intake and weight gain. In a trial designed to assess the effects of cisapride, Stacher et al. (1993) measured gastric emptying, gastric symptoms, and weight gain in 12 hospitalized patients with anorexia nervosa. In a 12-week trial, six patients were treated for 6 weeks with placebo and then switched to cisapride for 6 weeks, while the remaining six patients were treated with active medication for the entire 12-week period. Gastric emptying time improved in all patients, but those receiving the cisapride-cisapride sequence had shorter emptying times at the end of the study than those receiving the placebo-cisapride sequence. It also appeared that, at the end of the first 6 weeks, those who had received cisapride had fewer gastric complaints and greater increases in weight than those who had received placebo. However, the statistical significance of this difference was not reported. At the end of 12 weeks, medication offered no additional benefit on weight gain. Interpretation of this study is difficult because of the limited statistical data reported and very small sample size.

Szmukler et al. (1995) conducted a slightly shorter, randomized, controlled study with a larger sample size ($N = 29$) comparing the effect of cisapride (10 mg before meals) on gastric emptying time, gastrointestinal symptoms, and weight gain. In contrast to the previous study, they found no effect of medication on any measure, including gastric emptying time. The one exception was an increased perception of hunger in those who received cisapride, the meaning of which is unclear.

In summary, the effects of cisapride on the rate of gastric emptying in anorexia nervosa are, surprisingly, uncertain, and there is no convincing evidence supporting its routine use. However, for patients with severe gastrointestinal symptoms, a trial of cisapride may be worthwhile.

Zinc

The multiple vitamin and mineral abnormalities in anorexia nervosa caused by food restriction and poor nutrition, and the similarities in presentation between anorexia nervosa and zinc deficiency, including weight loss, alterations in taste and appetite, depression, and amenorrhea, prompted investigators to explore the role of zinc deficiency in anorexia nervosa (Bakan 1979, 1984). Case reports (Bryce-Smith and Simpson 1984; Esca et al. 1979; Thomsen 1978; Yamaguchi et al. 1992) and open (Safai-Kutti 1990) and controlled (Birmingham et al. 1994; Katz et al. 1987) trials of zinc supplementation have presented mixed results. In contrast to most of the other investigations of eating disorders, many of these studies were conducted in adolescents.

Safai-Kutti (1990) published the results of an open trial of zinc supplementation in a cohort of 20 young women (ages 14–26) meeting DSM-III-R criteria for anorexia nervosa. Of the 20 patients, 17 increased their body weight by 15% over the course of a follow-up period ranging from 8 to 56 months. Design of a double-blind study is described, but results have not yet been reported.

The results of three double-blind, placebo-controlled trials of zinc have been published. Katz and colleagues (1987) reported significantly lower levels of urinary zinc excretion in adolescent patients with anorexia nervosa compared to non-eating-disordered controls, suggesting zinc deficiency in the patients. Following supplementation, patients who received zinc scored significantly lower on measures of depression and anxiety. There was no significant effect on weight gain, however.

Birmingham et al. (1994) also published the results of a double-blind, placebo-controlled trial of zinc supplementation. Thirty-five female inpatients were randomized to receive either zinc gluconate (100 mg/day) or placebo until they showed a 10% increase in body mass index (BMI). Baseline plasma zinc levels were within normal limits and not significantly different between the two groups. The rate of increase in BMI was significantly faster in patients receiving daily zinc than those who received placebo ($P = .03$), and the authors suggest zinc supplementation may be helpful for augmenting weight gain in patients with anorexia nervosa.

Lask et al. (1993) reported the results of a double-blind, placebo-controlled 12-week trial of crossover design in patients with childhood-onset anorexia nervosa. Plasma zinc levels were evaluated in 26 hospitalized children who were subsequently randomized to receive 50 mg/day of zinc sulfate for 6 weeks and then placebo for 6 weeks or the reverse sequence. No significant difference was seen in rate of weight gain between zinc supplementation and placebo groups, and there was no evidence of a relationship between the baseline zinc level and benefit from zinc supplementation. The authors also noted that zinc levels rapidly returned to normal with refeeding and concluded that zinc supplementation was unnecessary.

One of the difficulties with the described studies is the lack of an accurate measure of zinc status (Hambidge 1988; Sandstead 1991). Serum levels of zinc may be normal in cases of mild but chronic zinc deficiency (Birmingham et al. 1994), and it has been suggested that "the best available indicator of zinc status is a favorable response to zinc supplementation" (Dinsmore et al. 1994, p. 253). Thus, the importance of zinc deficiency in the pathophysiology of anorexia nervosa is uncertain, and a role for zinc in the treatment of anorexia nervosa has not been clearly established.

Bulimia Nervosa

The development of pharmacological treatments for bulimia nervosa has been much more successful than for anorexia nervosa. Several factors have probably contributed to this difference. The prevalence of bulimia nervosa is roughly 10-fold higher than that of anorexia nervosa, and most patients can be treated on an outpatient basis. Both of these facts contribute to the relative ease and reduced costs of studies of bulimia nervosa relative to similar studies of anorexia nervosa. In addition, the medical condition of patients with bulimia nervosa is typically much less disturbed. Conceivably, this more normal physiological state may be necessary for the therapeutic impact of the psychotropic medications.

Anticonvulsants

Trials of medications in bulimia nervosa have been based on a variety of clinical models. With the notable exception of studies of antidepressant medications, discussed in a later section, trials of most medications have been few in number, small in sample size, and equivocal in outcome. For example, more than 20 years ago, the idea that patients with bulimia had a form of seizure disorder (Green and Rau 1974) prompted controlled studies of phenytoin (Wermuth et al. 1977) and carbamazepine (Kaplan et al. 1983). A robust response was not found, although there was a suggestion that a small number of patients might benefit.

Fenfluramine

Postulating that binge eating reflects an unrestrained appetite, several investigators have conducted trials of the appetite-suppressant *d*-fenfluramine. Results of a double-blind, placebo-controlled, crossover trial comparing desipramine to *d*-fenfluramine (Blouin et al. 1988) were favorable, with both drugs having

an effect on bingeing and purging. Those who received fenfluramine tended to fare slightly better. In contrast, Russell et al.
(1988) reported no significant benefit of *d*-fenfluramine over placebo, but their results were limited by a high dropout rate. In a
subsequent study from the same group, Fahy et al. (1993) examined the role of fenfluramine in patients receiving cognitive-
behavioral therapy and reported little additional benefit from
fenfluramine. That fenfluramine appears to have a limited effect
on the symptoms of bulimia nervosa is curious given the efficacy
of other serotonin-enhancing agents in the treatment of bulimia
nervosa (see later section) and the potency of fenfluramine in the
treatment of both obesity and binge-eating disorder (Stunkard et
al. 1996).

Antidepressants

Antidepressant agents appear far more powerful in curbing the
binge-purge cycle of bulimia nervosa than the other classes of
medication that have been studied. Clinical trials were initially
prompted by the observation of a high frequency of depressive
symptoms among patients with bulimia nervosa. Initial encouraging open trials of imipramine and phenelzine led to a series
of double-blind, placebo-controlled studies, utilizing parallel
and crossover designs, of various antidepressants (Agras et al.
1987; Enas et al. 1989; Horne et al. 1988; Hughes et al. 1986;
Mitchell and Groat 1984; Pope et al. 1983, 1989; Sabine et al.
1983; Walsh et al. 1988, 1991). With rare exception, these studies
found that antidepressant medication is superior to placebo in
the treatment of bulimia nervosa.

The optimum duration of pharmacologic treatment remains
an open question. In most of the controlled studies mentioned
earlier, the duration of treatment was relatively brief, generally
6–8 weeks, and few data are available on the long-term outcome
of pharmacological treatment. Pope et al. (1985) presented information on a group of patients 2 years after initial treatment with
imipramine. Although most patients remained improved at
follow-up, few continued on imipramine, and many had re-

quired multiple medication changes to maintain their response. Our own group (Walsh et al. 1991) reported that almost half of the patients who had initially responded to desipramine relapsed after 4 months despite continued desipramine therapy. Thus, while antidepressant medication can quickly induce a significant reduction in binge-purge frequency in most patients, it does not necessarily lead to lasting remission. This finding may signify the need for alternative or augmentation strategies such as the combination of medication and psychotherapy (see later section).

Another lingering question relates to optimum dose. In light of the high frequency of depressive symptoms seen in patients with bulimia nervosa, it is plausible that the effective dose for bulimia nervosa is identical to that for depression. It is also conceivable, however, that bulimia nervosa optimally responds to a different dose than does major depression. Only a single study of fluoxetine (Fluoxetine Bulimia Nervosa Collaborative Study Group 1992) has directly addressed this issue. In this large trial ($N = 387$), 129 patients with bulimia nervosa were randomly assigned to receive the standard dose of 20 mg/day, a second group of 129 patients received 60 mg/day, and a third group of 129 received placebo. The results showed that 20 mg/day of fluoxetine was, at most, marginally superior to placebo. On the other hand, 60 mg/day of fluoxetine was clearly superior. Subsequent studies of fluoxetine in bulimia nervosa have generally used 60 mg/day, which is usually tolerated with minimal side effects.

There is further evidence of a divergence between depression and bulimia nervosa. Although depressive symptoms and bulimia tend to co-occur, the presence of depressive symptoms does not predict the degree of improvement in bulimic symptoms with antidepressant treatment (Agras et al. 1987; Hughes et al. 1986; Walsh et al. 1988). That is, the eating disorder symptoms of patients with bulimia nervosa who are depressed do not respond more dramatically to antidepressant medication than do those of patients with bulimia nervosa who are not depressed. These data, and the preferential effectiveness of 60 mg/day, suggest that the mechanism of action of antidepressants in bulimia nervosa may be different from that in depression.

The pharmacological studies of bulimia nervosa have, for the most part, been restricted to normal-weight, adult women who purge through vomiting, and the results may not be generalizable to other populations including men, overweight patients, or patients with bulimia nervosa who use alternate methods of purging such as fasting or exercise. Unfortunately, whether these results are applicable to a younger, adolescent population also remains unclear.

Medication and Psychotherapy

Compelling data in the last decade have shown that forms of focused short-term psychotherapy, particularly cognitive-behavioral therapy (CBT), are effective in the treatment of bulimia nervosa (Wilson et al. 1997). Although undoubtedly a beneficial development, the existence of both pharmacotherapy and psychotherapy has complicated therapeutic recommendations, particularly because many important clinical questions cannot be answered directly with the controlled data available. For example, concerns regarding the comparative efficacy of medication and psychotherapy and, especially, regarding the long-term outcome of medication treatment leave the precise place of antidepressant medication in the treatment of bulimia nervosa unclear. The studies that have compared medication and psychotherapy and evaluated the potential benefits of combined treatment have yielded somewhat inconsistent results (Table 6–1).

To date, we are aware of seven randomized trials of combined treatment, not all of which have been placebo controlled. Various forms of psychotherapy have been employed, including nutritional counseling, individual psychotherapy (both cognitive behavioral and supportive), and group psychotherapy. The medications used have also varied, but all have been antidepressants. Earlier studies examined the benefit of TCAs, either imipramine

Table 6–1. Clinical trials in bulimia nervosa comparing psychotherapy, psychopharmacology, and combination therapy

Source of study	Design	N	Treatment groups	Duration of active treatment	Comment and conclusions
Mitchell et al. (1990)	Double-blind, randomized, placebo-controlled	174	IMI Placebo Group therapy + IMI Group therapy + placebo	8 weeks	Group treatment superior to medication alone Combined treatment significantly more effective only on measures of mood and anxiety
Fichter et al. (1991)	Double-blind, randomized, placebo-controlled	40	Inpatient psychotherapy + FLX Inpatient psychotherapy + placebo	5 weeks	Both groups improved, leading to possible ceiling effect Inpatient study; relevance to outpatient treatment unclear
Agras et al. (1992)	Randomized, assessor blinded	71	DMI for 16 weeks DMI for 24 weeks CBT and DMI for 16 weeks CBT and DMI for 24 weeks CBT	16, 24 weeks	CBT alone superior to DMI alone CBT and DMI for 24 weeks superior to CBT alone only on self-report measure of hunger or disinhibition
Leitenberg et al. (1994)	Randomized	21	DMI CBT CBT and DMI	20 weeks	Study terminated prematurely due to poor response to DMI and high dropout rate

Study	Design	N	Treatment	Duration	Results
Walsh et al. (1997)	Double-blind, randomized, placebo-controlled	120	DMI/FLX CBT and DMI/FLX CBT and placebo SPT and DMI/FLX SPT and placebo	16 weeks	CBT superior to SPT DMI/FLX superior to placebo CBT and DMI/FLX superior to CBT alone SPT and DMI/FLX no different from DMI/FLX alone Two-stage medication intervention (74% required medication change)
Goldbloom et al. (in press)	Randomized	76	FLX CBT CBT and FLX	16 weeks	Intent-to-treat analysis showed no difference between CBT and FLX and FLX alone Completer analysis showed CBT superior to FLX on reduction in subjective binge episodes Minimal difference between CBT alone and FLX alone Power of study limited by dropout rate
Beumont et al. (1997)	Double-blind, randomized, placebo-controlled	67	Nutritional counseling and FLX Nutritional counseling and placebo	8 weeks	FLX superior to placebo on measures of restraint, weight concern, and shape concern Differences did not persist at follow-up

Note. IMI, imipramine; FLX, fluoxetine; DMI, desimpramine; CBT, cognitive-behavioral therapy; SPT, supportive psychotherapy.

or desipramine, and more recent studies have used the SSRI fluoxetine because of its established efficacy and relatively few side effects.

Mitchell et al. (1990) published the first trial of the effect of combined medication and psychotherapy for the treatment of bulimia nervosa. Patients ($N = 174$) were randomly assigned to one of four treatment groups: placebo alone, imipramine alone, placebo and group psychotherapy, and imipramine and group psychotherapy. Outcome in each of the three active treatment groups was clearly superior to that in the placebo-only group. Patients receiving placebo and group psychotherapy, which was very structured, fared substantially better than did patients receiving only imipramine, indicating that the intensive group psychotherapy was superior to a course of imipramine. The combination of medication and group psychotherapy did not confer additional improvement in eating disorder symptoms, such as the frequencies of binge eating and purging over group psychotherapy alone. However, patients receiving imipramine—regardless of whether they also received group psychotherapy—had a significant reduction in symptoms of depression and anxiety compared to patients receiving placebo. Thus, there was some evidence, albeit limited, of an advantage for combining medication and psychotherapy.

Fichter and colleagues (1991), in Germany, examined the effect of fluoxetine (60 mg/day) compared with placebo in a population of patients hospitalized for bulimia nervosa who were actively engaged in a program of intensive behavioral psychotherapy. Although the study was not designed to address the efficacy of combined treatment, the authors explained their finding of no significant difference between the fluoxetine and placebo groups based on a "ceiling effect" of the psychotherapy. That is, the intensive inpatient psychotherapy was so effective that no additional medication effect could be observed.

Agras et al. (1992) compared individual CBT to a course of desipramine and to the combination of CBT and desipramine. Since the desipramine was given for either 16 or 24 weeks, this study had five treatment groups. One clear finding was that individual CBT was superior to treatment with medication alone.

The combination of desipramine and CBT was superior to CBT alone only on a single, self-report measure of hunger or disinhibition and only when desipramine treatment was continued for 24 weeks. This study suggested that individual CBT was superior to a single course of TCA and provided little evidence for an advantage of combining medication and psychotherapy, although the authors' recommendation was for combined treatment to offer the "broadest therapeutic benefits."

Leitenberg and colleagues (1994) attempted to study the interaction between desipramine and CBT but prematurely terminated the study because of a high dropout rate and unanticipated lack of response to desipramine alone.

Goldbloom et al. (in press) conducted a 16-week, randomized, controlled trial of individual CBT, fluoxetine, and the combination in 76 women with bulimia nervosa. All groups improved over the course of the study, and intent-to-treat analysis yielded no statistically significant differences in outcome. Completer analysis showed a significantly lower subjective binge frequency in the CBT-treated group compared with those taking fluoxetine alone. Interpretation of these data is limited by the absence of placebo and control groups and by a surprisingly high dropout rate (43%). It is uncertain whether the absence of differences in outcomes reflects similar treatment effects (i.e., that fluoxetine treatment is equivalent to CBT and that the combination is no better than either alone) or limited power to detect group differences.

Beumont et al. (1997) conducted a randomized, placebo-controlled trial of intensive nutritional counseling combined with fluoxetine. In an 8-week active treatment trial, with follow-up at 12 and 20 weeks, they compared 60 mg/day of fluoxetine to placebo in 67 patients receiving weekly nutritional counseling. Both the active medication and placebo groups showed improvement over the course of the study. During active treatment, fluoxetine was superior to placebo only on the measures of dietary restraint, weight concern, and shape concern. Although there were suggestions that bulimic symptoms reemerged after fluoxetine was discontinued, the fluoxetine- and placebo-treated groups had statistically similar levels of behavioral symptoms at both end of treatment and follow-up. Although this study suggests that fluoxetine does not dramatically add to the benefit of nutritional counseling, two concerns should be noted. First, the duration of medication intervention, 8 weeks, was relatively short. Second, the rate of improvement from nutritional counseling was quite impressive, with 61.5% of patients reporting no binge-eating episodes during the last week of active treatment. This degree of improvement may have limited the ability to detect an added medication effect.

Our group (Walsh et al. 1997) recently published the results of a placebo-controlled trial designed to compare two forms of psychotherapy for bulimia nervosa (individual CBT and individual supportive psychotherapy) and to examine the benefit of combining medication with psychotherapy. The medication intervention was unique in that it was two stage: patients randomized to receive active medication were first treated with desipramine; if they could not tolerate this medication or did not show sufficient improvement, they were switched to fluoxetine. The study was large (120 patients were randomized) and placebo controlled. The short-term results clearly document that CBT was superior to supportive psychotherapy and also indicate that the two-stage medication intervention modestly but significantly augmented the effect of psychotherapy. It was also of interest that the group of patients receiving only medication had a similar outcome on most measures to that of patients receiving CBT and placebo.

Although the results of these seven trials are by no means entirely consistent, they continue to emphasize that, in most patients, the symptoms of bulimia nervosa respond to both structured psychotherapeutic interventions and antidepressant medication. While early studies utilizing TCAs found that psychotherapy was clearly superior to medication alone, more recent studies, using fluoxetine and, in the Columbia study, a two-stage medication intervention, have not so clearly supported that superiority; however, it should be emphasized that lasting benefit of a time-limited intervention has been established *only* for structured psychotherapeutic interventions and not for medication alone. There are hints that combining medication and psychotherapy may confer some additional benefit, at least in the short term, but hard evidence for the superiority of combined treatment is limited. The most convincing data come from our own study, in which the effects of psychotherapy were not as dramatic as reported from other centers. Conceivably, it is easier to detect the additive benefit of medication in a population of patients relatively resistant to the effects of psychotherapy.

It is safe to conclude that we have at least three effective treatment strategies to employ in the treatment of bulimia nervosa: CBT alone, antidepressant medication alone, and combination therapy. Pressing questions for clinical research are how to match patients with treatments and what interventions are useful for the significant number of patients who fail to respond to these established treatments.

Practical Recommendations

Anorexia Nervosa

As reviewed previously, no pharmacological agent has been established to be of benefit in the treatment of anorexia nervosa. The mainstay of treatment is an eclectic approach, including psychological, nutritional, and behavioral elements aimed at restoring body weight and normalizing the distorted thinking concerning food, body shape, and weight. In addition, for children and adolescents with this disorder, involvement of the family in treatment is essential.

Antidepressant medications may be considered when evidence of a significant mood disturbance or of obsessive-compulsive disorder persists or emerges after weight restoration. Because of its side effect profile, extensive experience in the treatment of bulimia nervosa, and more limited experience in anorexia nervosa, fluoxetine is probably the preferred agent. Treatment may be initiated at 10–20 mg/day. If target symptoms include obsessive-compulsive disorder, higher doses (e.g., 60 mg/day) should be employed and can be reached for most patients over 1–2 weeks. The limited data available suggest that fluoxetine can be used safely for patients with anorexia nervosa, but the physiological disturbances associated with this disorder merit careful monitoring of medication side effects and interactions. It is likely that other SSRIs have similar therapeutic effects, but there is essentially no published information concerning their use in anorexia nervosa.

Antipsychotic medications may rarely be considered for symptom control in particularly refractory patients. Because its sedating properties have been thought to be useful, chlorpromazine has been used in small doses, usually beginning at 25 mg/day. However, the risks of this class of agents need to be carefully weighed and the physical effects, such as lowering of blood pressure, monitored. These cautions are especially relevant in the child and adolescent populations. The newer atypical antipsychotic agents (e.g., olanzapine) may offer an improved side effect profile, but no information is currently available on their use in anorexia nervosa. Cisapride, 10 mg taken 30 minutes before meals, may be considered for patients with severe complaints of gastric fullness or bloating; the clinician should be mindful, however, that such symptoms improve with refeeding.

Bulimia Nervosa

The major pharmacological intervention to consider for patients with bulimia nervosa is the use of an antidepressant. Because it has been extensively studied and because information concerning the effective dose is available, fluoxetine should be considered the drug of first choice. The preferred dose is 60 mg/day; most patients of normal weight with bulimia nervosa can be started immediately on this amount or can increase from 20 to 60 mg/day over the course of a week. Side effects are rarely a major problem. Anecdotal information suggests that other SSRIs are probably also effective and should be considered if the use of fluoxetine is complicated by the need for other medications with which it may interact.

In closing, it should be reemphasized that the data on the use of psychotropic medications for eating disorders have been obtained almost entirely from studies of adults. It is not known whether children and adolescents with these disorders have similar responses. As in the case of other psychiatric disorders of childhood and adolescence, this is a fertile area for future research.

References

Agras WS, Dorian B, Kirkley BG, et al: Imipramine in the treatment of bulimia: a double-blind controlled study. International Journal of Eating Disorders 6:29–38, 1987

Agras WS, Rossiter EM, Arnow B, et al: Pharmacologic and cognitive-behavioral treatment for bulimia nervosa: a controlled comparison. Am J Psychiatry 149:82–87, 1992

American Psychiatric Association: Practice guidelines for eating disorders. Am J Psychiatry 150:207–228, 1993

Attia, EA, Haiman C, Walsh BT, et al: Does fluoxetine augment the inpatient treatment of anorexia nervosa? Am J Psychiatry (in press)

Bakan R: The role of zinc in anorexia nervosa: etiology and treatment. Med Hypotheses 5:731–736, 1979

Bakan R: Anorexia and zinc. Lancet 2:874, 1984

Barry VC, Klawans HL: On the role of dopamine in the pathophysiology of anorexia nervosa. J Neural Transm Gen Sect 38:107–122, 1976

Beumont PJV, Russell J, Touyz S, et al: Intensive nutritional counselling in bulimia nervosa: a role for supplementation with fluoxetine? Aust N Z J Psychiatry 31:514–524, 1997

Biederman J, Herzog DB, Rivinus TM, et al: Amitriptyline in the treatment of anorexia nervosa: a double-blind, placebo-controlled study. J Clin Psychopharmacol 5:10–16, 1985

Birmingham CL, Goldner EM, Bakan R: Controlled trial of zinc supplementation in anorexia nervosa. International Journal of Eating Disorders 15:251–255, 1994

Blouin AG, Blouin JH, Perez EL, et al: Treatment of bulimia with fenfluramine and desipramine. J Clin Psychopharmacol 8:261–269, 1988

Bryce-Smith D, Simpson R: Case of anorexia nervosa responding to zinc sulphate (letter). Lancet 2:350, 1984

Dally P, Sargant W: A new treatment of anorexia nervosa. BMJ 1:1770–1773, 1960

Dally P, Sargant W: Treatment and outcome of anorexia nervosa. BMJ 2:793–795, 1966

Dinsmore WW, McMaster D, Alderice JT: Zinc and anorexia nervosa. International Journal of Eating Disorders 15:251–255, 1994

Enas GG, Pope HG, Levine LR: Fluoxetine in bulimia nervosa: double blind study, in New Research Program and Abstracts: American Psychiatric Association 142nd Annual Meeting, San Francisco, May 6–11, 1989, p 204

Esca SA, Brenner W, Mach K, et al: Kwashiorkor-like zinc deficiency syndrome in anorexia nervosa. Acta Dermato-Venereologia (Stockholm) 59:361–364, 1979

Fahy TA, Eisler I, Russell GFM: A placebo-controlled trial of *d*-fenfluramine in bulimia nervosa. Br J Psychiatry 162:597–603, 1993

Ferguson JM: Treatment of an anorexia nervosa patient with fluoxetine (letter). Am J Psychiatry 144:1239, 1987

Fichter MM, Leibl K, Rief W, et al: Fluoxetine versus placebo: a double-blind study with bulimic inpatients undergoing intensive psychotherapy. Pharmacopsychiatry 24:1–7, 1991

Fluoxetine Bulimia Nervosa Collaborative Study Group: Fluoxetine in the treatment of bulimia nervosa: a multicenter, placebo-controlled, double-blind trial. Arch Gen Psychiatry 49:139–147, 1992

Garner DM, Garfinkel PE (eds): Handbook of Treatment for Eating Disorders. New York, Guilford, 1997

Goldberg SC, Halmi KA, Eckert ED, et al: Cyproheptadine in anorexia nervosa. Br J Psychiatry 134:67–70, 1979

Goldbloom DS, Olmsted M, Davis R, et al: A randomized controlled trial of fluoxetine and cognitive behavioral therapy for bulimia nervosa: short-term outcome. Behav Res Ther (in press)

Green RS, Rau JH: Treatment of compulsive eating disturbances with anticonvulsant medication. Am J Psychiatry 131:428–432, 1974

Gross HA, Ebert MH, Faden VB, et al: A double-blind controlled trial of lithium carbonate in primary anorexia nervosa. J Clin Psychopharmacol 1:376–381, 1981

Gross HA, Ebert MH, Faden VB, et al: A double-blind trial of $\Delta 9$-tetrahydrocannabinol in primary anorexia nervosa. J Clin Psychopharmacol 3:165–171, 1983

Gwirtsman HE, Guze BH, Yager J, et al: Fluoxetine treatment of anorexia nervosa: an open clinical trial. J Clin Psychiatry 51:378–382, 1990

Halmi KA, Eckert ED, LaDu TJ, et al: Anorexia nervosa: treatment efficacy of cyproheptadine and amitriptyline. Arch Gen Psychiatry 43:177–181, 1986

Hambidge KM: Assessing the trace element status of man. Proc Nutr Soc 47:37–44, 1988

Horne RL, Ferguson JM, Pope HG, et al: Treatment of bulimia with bupropion: a multicenter controlled trial. J Clin Psychiatry 49:262–266, 1988

Hughes PL, Wells LA, Cunningham CJ: The dexamethasone suppression test in bulimia before and after successful treatment with desipramine. J Clin Psychiatry 47:515–517, 1986

Kaplan AS, Garfinkel PE, Darby PL, et al: Carbamazepine in the treatment of bulimia. Am J Psychiatry 140:1225–1226, 1983

Katz RL, Keen CL, Litt IF, et al: Zinc deficiency in anorexia nervosa. Journal of Adolescent Health Care 8:400–406, 1987

Kaye WH, Weltzin TE, Hsu G, et al: Relapse prevention with fluoxetine in anorexia nervosa: a double-blind placebo-controlled study. 150th American Psychiatric Association Meeting, San Diego, CA, May 17, 1997

Lacey JH, Crisp AH: Hunger, food intake, and weight: the impact of clomipramine on a refeeding anorexia nervosa population. Postgrad Med J 56(suppl 1):79–85, 1980

Lask B, Fosson A, Rolfe U, et al: Zinc deficiency and childhood-onset anorexia nervosa. J Clin Psychiatry 54:63–66, 1993

Leitenberg H, Rosen JC, Wolf J, et al: Comparison of cognitive-behavioral therapy and desipramine in the treatment of bulimia nervosa. Behav Res Ther 32:37–45, 1994

Mitchell JE, Groat R: A placebo-controlled, double-blind trial of amitriptyline in bulimia. J Clin Psychopharmacol 4:186–193, 1984

Mitchell JE, Pyle RL, Eckert ED, et al: A comparison study of antidepressants and structured group psychotherapy in the treatment of bulimia nervosa. Arch Gen Psychiatry 47:149–157, 1990

Pope HG, Hudson JI, Jonas JM, et al: Bulimia treated with imipramine: a placebo-controlled, double-blind study. Am J Psychiatry 140:554–558, 1983

Pope HG Jr, Hudson JI, Jonas JM, et al: Antidepressant treatment of bulimia: a two-year follow-up study. J Clin Psychopharmacol 5:320–327, 1985

Pope HG Jr, Keck PEJ, McElroy SL, et al: A placebo-controlled study of trazodone in bulimia nervosa. J Clin Psychopharmacol 9:254–259, 1989

Russell GFM, Checkley SA, Feldman J, et al: A controlled trial of d-fenfluramine in bulimia nervosa. Clin Neuropharmacol 11(suppl 1):S146–S159, 1988

Sabine EJ, Yonace A, Farrington AJ, et al: Bulimia nervosa: a placebo controlled double-blind therapeutic trial of mianserin. Br J Clin Pharmacol 15:195S–202S, 1983

Safai-Kutti S: Oral zinc supplementation in anorexia nervosa. Acta Psychiatr Scand Suppl 361:14–17, 1990

Sandstead H: Assessment of zinc nutriture. J Lab Clin Med 118:299–300, 1991

Stacher G, Abatzi-Wenzel TA, Wiesnagrotzki S, et al: Gastric emptying, body weight, and symptoms in primary anorexia nervosa: long term effects of cisapride. Br J Psychiatry 162:398–402, 1993

Strober M, Freeman R, DeAntonio M, et al: Does adjunctive fluoxetine influence the post-hospital course of anorexia nervosa? a 24-month prospective, longitudinal follow-up, and comparison with historical controls. Psychopharmacol Bull (in press)

Stunkard A, Berkowitz R, Tanrikut C, et al: *d*-Fenfluramine treatment of binge eating disorder. Am J Psychiatry 153:1455–1459, 1996

Szmukler GI, Young GP, Miller G, et al: A controlled trial of cisapride in anorexia nervosa. International Journal of Eating Disorders 17:347–357, 1995

Thomsen K: Zinc, liver cirrhosis, and anorexia nervosa. Acta-Dermato Venereologia (Stockholm) 59:361–364, 1978

Vandereycken W: Neuroleptics in the short-term treatment of anorexia nervosa: a double-blind placebo-controlled study with sulpiride. Br J Psychiatry 144:288–292, 1984

Vandereycken W, Pierloot R: Pimozide combined with behavior therapy in the short-term treatment of anorexia nervosa. Acta Psychiatr Scand 66:445–450, 1982

Vigersky RA, Loriaux DL: The effect of cyproheptadine in anorexia nervosa: a double-blind trial, in Anorexia Nervosa. Edited by Vigersky RA. New York, Raven, 1977, pp 349–356

Walsh BT, Gladis M, Roose SP, et al: Phenelzine vs. placebo in 50 patients with bulimia. Arch Gen Psychiatry 45:471–475, 1988

Walsh BT, Hadigan CM, Devlin MJ, et al: Long-term outcome of antidepressant treatment for bulimia nervosa. Am J Psychiatry 148:1206–1212, 1991

Walsh BT, Wilson GT, Loeb KL, et al: Medication and psychotherapy in the treatment of bulimia nervosa. Am J Psychiatry 154:523–531, 1997

Wermuth BM, Davis KL, Hollister LE, et al: Phenytoin treatment of the binge-eating syndrome. Am J Psychiatry 134:1249–1253, 1977

Wilens TE, Biederman J, Baldessarini RJ, et al: Cardiovascular effects of therapeutic doses of tricyclic antidepressants in children and adolescents. J Am Acad Child Adolesc Psychiatry 35:1491–1501, 1996

Wilson GT, Fairburn CG, Agras WS: Cognitive-behavioral therapy for bulimia nervosa, in Handbook of Treatment for Eating Disorders. Edited by Garner DM, Garfinkel PE. New York, Guilford, 1997, pp 67–93

Yamaguchi H, Arita Y, Hara Y, et al: Anorexia nervosa responding to zinc supplementation: a case report. Gastroenterologia Japonica 27:554–558, 1992

Afterword

B. Timothy Walsh, M.D.

The six chapters in this text have provided a timely overview of a field in rapid development. Within the last year, the National Institute of Mental Health (NIMH) has established research units in pediatric psychopharmacology to spur the evaluation of psychopharmacological interventions for children and adolescents, and President Clinton has called on the Food and Drug Administration (FDA) to augment its examination of new drugs likely to be prescribed in the pediatric age range. These developments portend a dramatic increase in the research database underlying pediatric psychopharmacology in the next several years.

I hope the information and the perspectives in these chapters not only provide practical guidance for clinicians but also serve as an introduction to one of the most immediately interesting areas in all of psychiatry. And, in closing, I wish to thank the contributors to this text for providing a superb introduction to this important and exciting field.

Index

Page numbers in **boldface** type refer to tables.

loxapine, 75
olanzapine, 77, 79–81, 83–84
risperidone, 77–78
side effects, 75–76
nonschizophrenia disorders, 68–70
schizophrenia, childhood-onset
cause, 66–67
diagnosis, 67–68
education about, 71–72
neuroleptic-nonresponsive, 76
practical advice for, 72
treatment of, 70–74
maintenance, 81–83

Risperidone
for bipolar disorder, 107
for psychotic disorders, 77–78

Selective mutism, 118–119
Selective serotonin reuptake
inhibitors (SSRIs)
for ADHD, 56
for anorexia nervosa, 153–154
for anxiety disorders, 129–134
for OCD, 19–21
Separation anxiety disorder, 116–117
Sertraline, for OCD, 19–21
Social phobia and selective mutism,
118–119
Stimulants
for ADHD, 34–36, 46–47, 51–53
dosage, 40–42
efficacy, 36–39, 42–43
extended-release forms, 49
long-term, 43, 48–49
side effects, 49–51
stimulant choice, 42
for ADHD with tic disorders,
12–14
Streptococcal infections,
neuropsychiatric disorders
and, 5
Sulpiride for anorexia nervosa,
151–152
Sydenham's chorea, 5

TCAs. *See* Tricyclic antidepressants
Tetrahydrocannabinol, for anorexia
nervosa, 156–157
Thymoleptics, for bipolar disorders,
104
carbamazepine, 106, 107
gabapentin, 106
lamotrigine, 106
lithium carbonate, 104–105, 107,
107
valproate (divalproex sodium),
105–106, 107, **107**
Tic disorders
ADHD and, treatment of, **7**, 9–17
age and, 9
comorbidity, 1, 3
definitions, 1–2
etiology, 4–5
immune-mediated, 4–5
medications for, **7**, 8–9, 9
clonidine, 9–10, 13
guanfacine, 10
neuroleptics, 14–17
prevalence, 2
Tourette's syndrome
with or without ADHD, treatment
of, **7**, 9–17
definition, 1–2
treatment of, 8–9
Transient tic disorder, definition, 2
Tricyclic antidepressants (TCAs)
for ADHD, 54
for anorexia nervosa, 152–153
for anxiety disorders, 139–142
for tic disorders and ADHD,
10–12

Valproate (divalproex sodium), for
bipolar disorders, 105–106,
107, **107**
Venlafaxine, for ADHD, 55–56

Zinc, for anorexia nervosa, 158–159